DARCEY BUSSELL'S
DANCE
BODY
WORKOUT

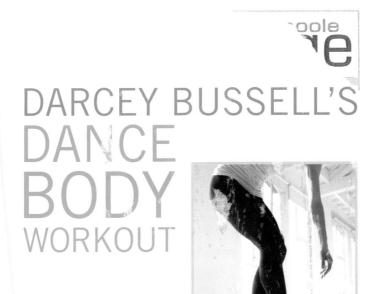

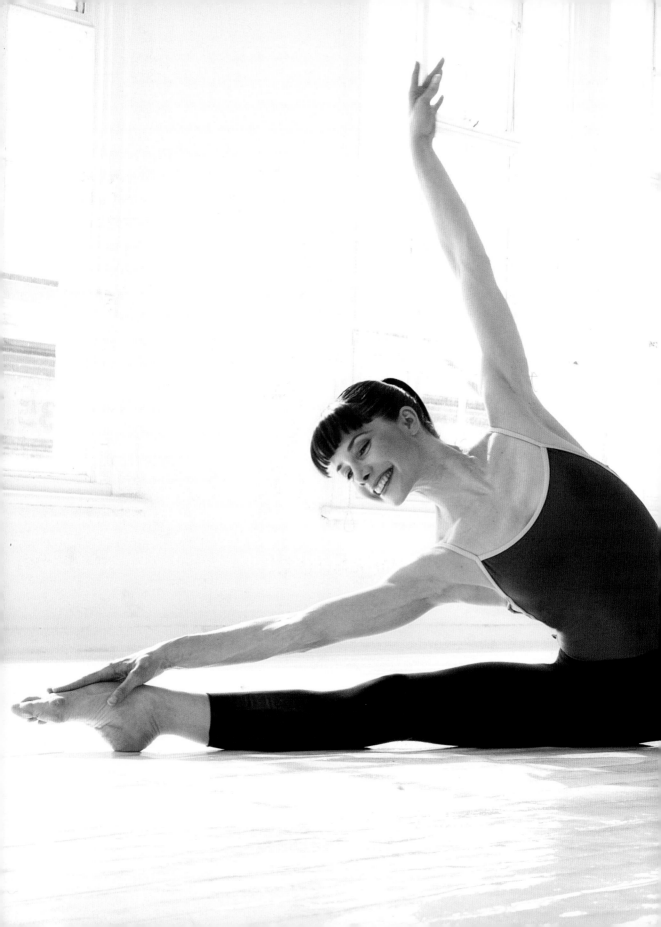

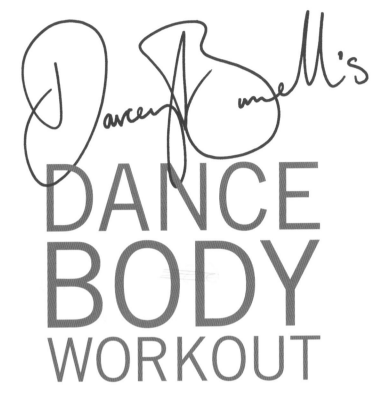

Darcey Bussell's
DANCE
BODY
WORKOUT

Tone · Sculpt · Stretch

MICHAEL JOSEPH
an imprint of penguin books

To my family, and especially James and Jo.

WARNING

If you have any medical condition, are pregnant or suffer from back problems, the exercises described in this book should not be followed without first consulting your doctor or seeking expert advice. All guidelines and warnings should be read carefully and the author and publishers cannot accept responsibility for injuries or damage arising out of failure to do so.

MICHAEL JOSEPH

Published by the Penguin Group

Penguin Books Ltd, 80 Strand, London WC2R 0RL, England

Penguin Group (USA) Inc., 375 Hudson Street, New York, New York 10014, USA

Penguin Group (Canada), 90 Eglinton Avenue East, Suite 700, Toronto, Ontario, Canada M4P 2Y3 (a division of Pearson Penguin Canada Inc.)

Penguin Ireland, 25 St Stephen's Green, Dublin 2, Ireland (a division of Penguin Books Ltd)

Penguin Group (Australia), 250 Camberwell Road, Camberwell, Victoria 3124, Australia (a division of Pearson Australia Group Pty Ltd)

Penguin Books India Pvt Ltd, 11 Community Centre, Panchsheel Park, New Delhi – 110 017, India

Penguin Group (NZ), 67 Apollo Drive, Mairangi Bay, Auckland 1310, New Zealand (a division of Pearson New Zealand Ltd)

Penguin Books (South Africa) (Pty) Ltd, 24 Sturdee Avenue, Rosebank, Johannesburg 2196, South Africa

Penguin Books Ltd, Registered Offices: 80 Strand, London WC2R 0RL, England

www.penguin.com

First published 2007
1

Copyright © Darcey Bussell, 2007

Photography by Iain Philpott

Set in Berkley and Trade Gothic
Colour reproduction by Dot Gradations Ltd, UK
Made and printed in Italy by Printer Trento

A CIP catalogue record for this book is available from the British Library

ISBN: 978-0-718-14767-9

CONTENTS

INTRODUCTION

I love my life, but as any working mother knows, it's not always easy to be a mother and manage a career. I've now been dancing professionally for nearly twenty years and have danced for some of the most exciting companies in the world, such as the Royal Ballet, the New York City Ballet and the Kirov Ballet of St. Petersburg, but I also have two daughters, and this means I am constantly juggling.

Like anyone who does the same, I've learnt that the only way to stay sane and make it all work is to be prepared in every aspect of my daily life, whether this is memorizing my performance timetable, working out what is and isn't in the fridge or delegating who's picking up the girls from school every day. Being organized like this sounds fanatical, but it works for me. The upside is that I am calm at work and at home and that, in turn, helps keep my girls calm and happy.

Of course I'd be lying if I didn't admit there are times when I feel exhausted. The hardest part of the year for me is always the end of season, when I am physically most tired, but I am lucky because I have a great PA and a fantastic support team. I know I can delegate tasks, which makes my life easier and also gets me some time for myself, even if it's just five minutes alone in the bath. And as hard as it may be, I absolutely adore being a mother and watching my girls grow. Phoebe, who is five years old now, loves to watch me do class and recently even sat through a whole two-and-a-half-hour ballet performance (with breaks). She loved the dance, but for her it was the atmosphere in the auditorium, the lights going

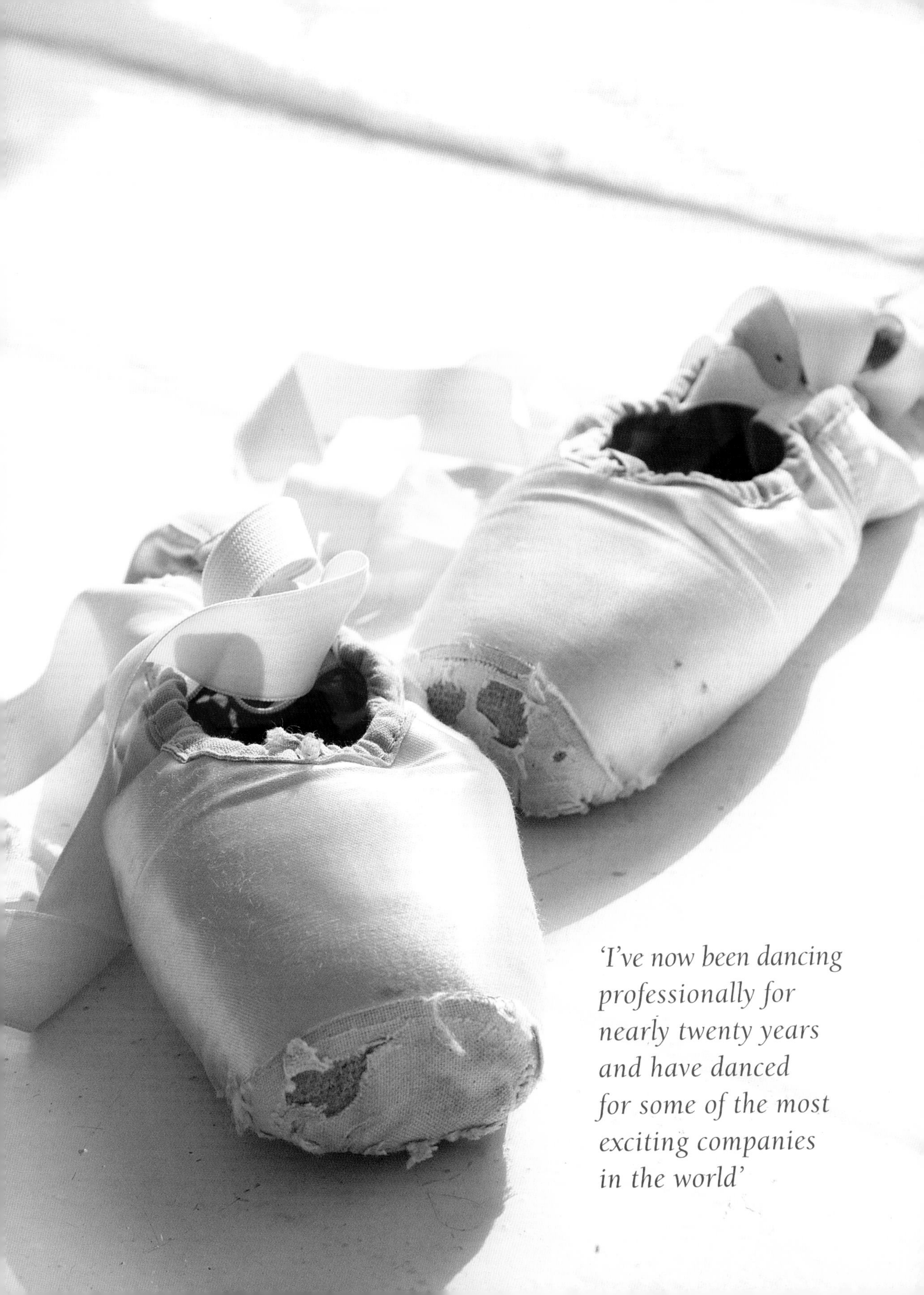

'I've now been dancing
professionally for
nearly twenty years
and have danced
for some of the most
exciting companies
in the world'

down and, especially, how many outfits I was wearing in the performance that made it so exciting.

Like Phoebe, I have always loved everything about dance, but at her age I certainly never fantasized about being a ballerina, and no one would ever have said that I was born to dance. As a child I was always more athletic and had that kind of body, though as I've got older and have had kids, I've become more sinewy. Now I certainly couldn't imagine my world without ballet because it's become my natural element.

I love to dance because it makes me feel free. Like swimming, you are working every single part of your body as you move and it's an amazing feeling. I also love the addictive sensation of perfecting a dance movement – the whole process of working really hard to get a technique absolutely right. I always feel if you're watching a dancer and can still see the shapes of the movements in the air when they've stopped, you know they've done it well, and that's the perfection I aim for.

I wrote this book because I wanted to create a workout that highlights this aspect of my work and shows how the precision and intricacy of ballet exercises can shape your body. Ballet exercises, contrary to popular opinion, are not just for ballet dancers; they are a method for anybody to strengthen and lengthen their body. The Pilates, floor barre and stretch combination workout is the best way I can give you a feel of what it's like to work out like a dancer. The exercises differ greatly to your standard gym exercises simply because our aim is different to that of other athletes. We have to keep our bodies both lean and powerful and, to do this, we need to work on building muscle strength without bulking up. The focus is on lengthening and toning above everything else. It may sound easier than what you've been used to, but you will be surprised at the intensity of it all.

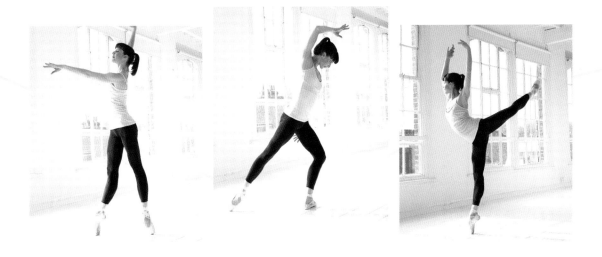

I remember doing the floor barre (a ballet workout that's performed on the floor instead of at the barre) from the age of twelve years. It really helped strengthen my body and from that I moved on to Pilates. I still do barre work for thirty minutes a day, six days a week, because as any dancer knows, barre work is essential and you really can't dance without it, though it is only the beginning of a full dancer's class, which is part of our day. Pilates is also one of my exercise mainstays and the technique that helped me regain my form after the birth of my daughters. It is these two elements, Pilates and dance, together with regular stretching, that I know helps me remain strong enough to be a professional dancer to this day.

Do the programme regularly and you'll reap countless benefits for your body such as better poise, a flatter stomach and increased muscle tone and strength, to name but a few. Best of all, the combination of Pilates, floor barre and stretch will help you to become more aware of your body and how you use it in everyday life. Do the programme at least three times a week and it will not only help your body to feel more flexible and strong, but will also give you a small taste of what it's like to be a ballet dancer, without actually having to dance.

Darcey

A UNIQUE WORKOUT – PILATES, FLOOR BARRE AND STRETCH

If you've ever seen a ballet dancer in action, you'll know that despite the athletic and vigorous nature of ballet these days, dancers are far from being muscle bound and burly. This is because ballet, unlike other workouts, does not bulk up the body, but rather defines and sculpts it. This means that while dancers are undoubtedly physically powerful and able-bodied, we do not look overdeveloped and large like other types of athletes. This is important for us because ballet naturally calls for us to look light and graceful as we dance, so the way we exercise and work on our bodies has to reflect this.

This is just one reason why ballet and its associated workouts offer such a unique and powerful advantage when it comes to exercising. Use this type of body conditioning and it will enable you to become not only stronger, but also leaner, more defined and supple than if you, say, work out at the gym. If you are secretly someone who has a longing to dance, or even the desire to join an adult ballet class, this workout can also give you a taster of how ballet can affect your body positively. However, don't dismiss this plan if ballet is the furthest thing from your mind, because the Pilates, floor barre and stretch programme is a powerful workout that can help anyone feel fitter and stronger, no matter if you're a beginner or a seasoned athlete. Follow the workout in its entirety three times a week and it will help chisel your body, improve your posture, as well as increase your range of movement and build shape and definition to your muscles.

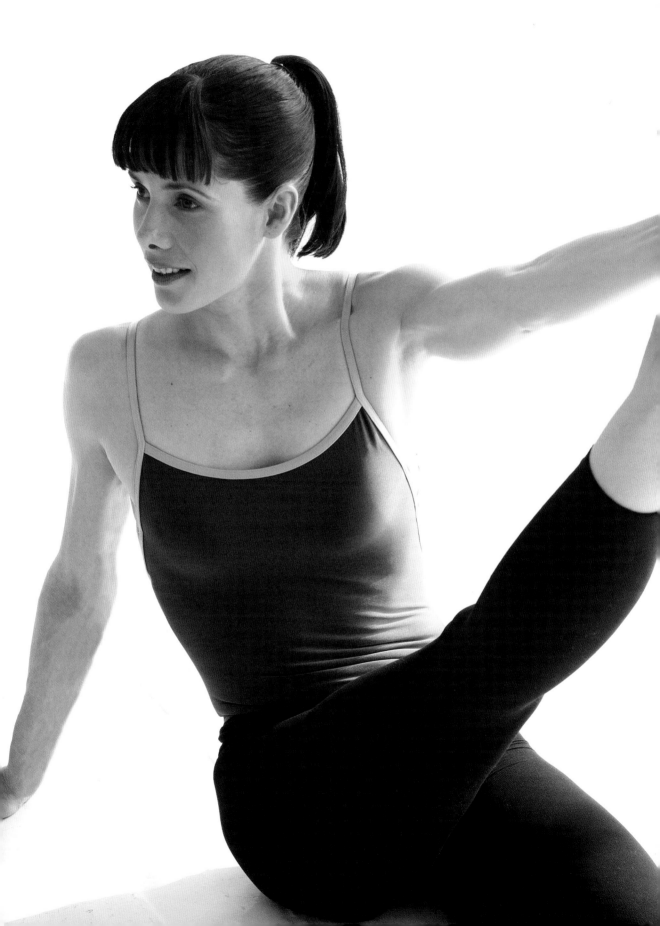

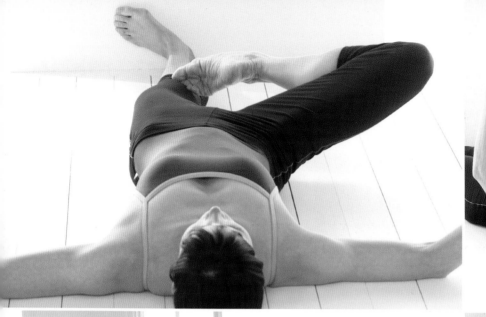

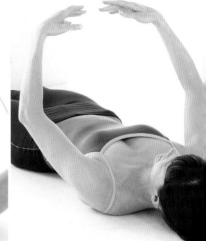

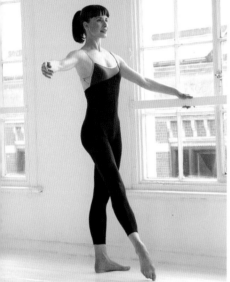

'We do barre work because it helps prepare us to stand and dance unsupported and we do it six days a week, every week, of our careers to help keep our bodies in shape'

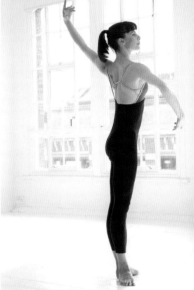

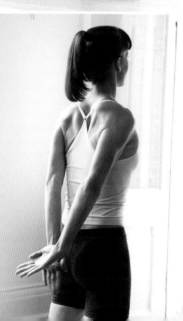

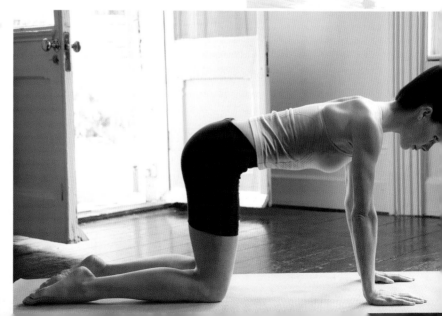

Of course, most non-dancers (and even some dancers) are intimidated by the thought of ballet and ballet-style exercises, thinking that if they didn't start dancing as a child, or if they don't have natural coordination and a classic ballet body, ballet exercises will be of no use to them. This isn't true: barre exercises can be done by anyone of any shape and they are an ideal way to get fit without placing too much strain on the body. Better still, with the floor barre you do not need to have previous knowledge of ballet, because the exercises are designed to be accessible. This means that you can tone your muscles and strengthen your body no matter what your previous experience of dance, or even working out, is.

All the exercises in the Pilates, floor barre and stretch programme focus their attention on lengthening the muscles while making them strong. The floor barre itself is based on the daily ballet workout that is usually performed by dancers standing up at the barre (the wooden rail you'll find alongside a mirror in any ballet studio). We do barre work because it helps prepare us to stand and dance unsupported and we do it six days a week, every week, of our careers to help keep our bodies in shape. This series, however, has been adapted to the floor for a number of reasons. Firstly, performing the exercises while lying down will help non-dancers to achieve many of the benefits that dancers get from ballet, without having to worry about stability. The floor gives perfect support and prevents you having to think about your centre of gravity changing and/or losing your balance as you execute the leg lifts and raises. Secondly, lying down helps protect your back from injury, while allowing you to reach and find a greater range of movement than you would have standing up. And thirdly, it will give you a better chance of doing all the exercises correctly.

As a progression, for anyone who is eager to get the feel of what it's like to do a professional dancer's standing barre, at the end of the workout programme is a short standing programme which, while less complicated than the usual barre workout, will give you a good idea of what the exercises feel like without the support of the floor.

All the barre exercises will work your body in ways it has never been worked before by asking you not only to focus on specific muscle groups, but also to concentrate on elongating your body and holding it from its core (your stomach). You will probably also discover new or underused muscles. On first glance, the workout may seem repetitious, but this is the way ballet is taught. The body learns by repetition and so the more you do something, the easier it will be to remember it and the faster it will click into place. For this reason, the floor barre starts out with slow moves and gradually advances on to faster and more complicated ones. The repetition also warms up every joint and muscle. Your goal, therefore, should be not to quickly gravitate to the centre (what dancers call the middle of the room) and hope to perform elaborate jumps, but to work on improving your flexibility and suppleness so you can look leaner and carry yourself better in your everyday life without having to think about it.

To achieve this, you need to start from scratch. One of the things I quickly learnt about ballet class is that there really is a reason for every exercise.

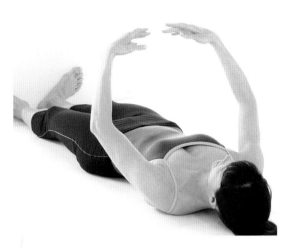

This is because there is no point in spending time on exercises that don't help us to become better dancers or achieve the right kind of muscle tone. As a result, every exercise in this workout (and in any ballet workout) has a definite reason and purpose. For instance, the *pliés* (knee bends), with which the exercises begin, do seem simple but are a crucial part of the whole workout. This is because when you do a *plié*, the muscles of the thigh contract, expand and warm up. Bring in a *tendu* (a brushing movement of the foot) and the thigh needs to work as the tendons and muscles of the foot start to activate. This then builds to the next exercise, and so on and so on. However difficult you find the workout at first, do persevere because a few weeks into the programme you will definitely notice a stronger, flatter stomach, better posture and the beginnings of a more defined look to your legs and arms.

Overall, you'll find that the floor barre is perfect for body conditioning because it targets the abdominals, the glutes, thighs, calves and arms, and all while giving you an idea of how ballet dancers exercise. It means you will work your stomach as you firm your thighs, lift your bottom and streamline your legs. This is because ballet itself is not static, so neither are the exercises. All the exercises work in opposition to each other; for example, if one leg raises up, the other counteracts the movement by working the opposite way so that muscles are always in motion. This helps you to achieve core stability and the poise dancers are known for.

The floor barre, therefore, has a unique extra aspect in that it can also help you become aware of how you hold and use your body in everyday life. If you sit slumped over a computer or desk every day or spend your time looking down at the pavement as you walk, this workout will give you the deportment of

'Pilates is also just the thing for non-dancers looking to tone up and learn how to use their bodies because, apart from strengthening the muscles, it will also give you a real sense of your body and how it moves'

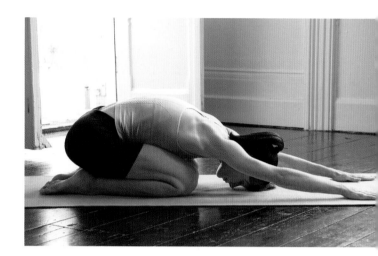

a dancer by reminding you to hold your head high and maintain your posture at all times. The exercises will also teach you how to hold yourself from your stomach, so no matter what you're doing – shopping, lifting children or running for the bus – you'll be able to use your body without twisting it out of alignment or putting strain on your back and hurting yourself.

The floor barre has been brought together here with Pilates and stretch for a number of reasons. Firstly, this combination is essentially the central part of any dancer's exercise programme. Secondly, the three elements work fantastically well together because they all focus on building strength and creating length through the body. Thirdly, as anyone who read my first book *Pilates for Life* will know, I adore Pilates. I've been doing the technique since I left school and, twenty years later, I still love the effect it has on my body and mind. It's an amazing exercise technique, but for me Pilates is also a lifesaver because it's the method that helped me regain my form after I had foot surgery for ankle spurs in 1994 and once again in 2003. It also helped me get back into shape after the birth of my daughters, Phoebe in 2001 and Zoe in 2004.

If you've yet to hear about Pilates, it's essentially a unique method of body conditioning that was developed nearly a hundred years ago in Germany by Joseph H. Pilates. He initially developed the technique to strengthen his body after suffering from rickets as a child, but went on to teach it to fellow internees in a prisoner of war camp during the First World War and later, in the 1920s, set up a studio in New York and taught it to dancers such as Martha Graham and George Balanchine. Unlike other body techniques, it's become a favourite of dancers because it works on strengthening, lengthening and toning muscles (rather than building and bulking them) and so helps create a perfect lean and long look, which is ideal for dancers.

Pilates is also just the thing for non-dancers looking to tone up and learn how to use their bodies because, apart from strengthening the muscles, it will also give you a real sense of your body and how it moves. This is just one reason why numerous athletes, actors and performers love it and why I have created a Pilates warm up programme as a precursor to the floor barre. Doing Pilates as a warm up will not only help you to reach a full range of movement in the floor barre, but also help you to get used to moving your body in the way that dancers do, as well as help you to focus your concentration and connect your mind and body. This means you need to pay constant attention to how you execute and perform the exercises, something that's crucial throughout the whole of this workout.

The final component of stretch exercises is something that every single workout programme, from football to ice-skating, should contain. Dancers of all ages and experience know the importance and value of stretching, which is why if you wander around any ballet studio, you're always guaranteed to see dancers stretching in corridors, at the barre and really anywhere they can find a space. We stretch to help keep our bodies flexible and supple and to keep our muscles from becoming tight. For a dancer, this is as important as dancing and barre work because without it, we are likely to get injured. For non-dancers, it's even more important because over time our muscles naturally become stiff and painful and the more inactive we are, the sorer we will become, which not only limits our range of movement but also increases our chance of an injury.

Stretching will not only help keep your muscles loose, but also improve your flexibility, which means you can do things like bend down without feeling a twinge in your back or turn suddenly without feeling a sharp pain in your body. Sadly, of late, stretching has got a bad press and lots of people now assume that it has no real use and so either rush through their stretches or assume it's okay to skip stretching completely. This is wrong for a number of reasons. Firstly, research shows that it's not beneficial to stretch before warming up and this is true because the muscles need to be warm before you attempt to put them through a range of movement. For this reason, I have made stretching the cool down part of this programme and Pilates the warm up. Secondly, stretching is essential if you have been through a rigorous workout and don't want to end up with aches and pains caused by lactic acid build up in the muscle tissue (stretching helps release the build up of these toxins). This, in turn, will enable you to work out again sooner. Thirdly, stretching every day will help lengthen tight, short muscles, which are a major factor in dance, sport and everyday injuries.

Staying flexible can also help you improve and maintain your balance, boost your overall energy and improve your posture. These are just some of the reasons why ballet workouts, Pilates and yoga have become so popular of late. So whatever your goal is in doing this workout programme, make stretching an essential part of the equation. If all of the above doesn't convince you to stretch, then think about this: stretching your muscles enables you to extend your body to its fullest range of movement, which then helps you to look taller and appear instantly leaner. Plus, it releases stress and tension in the body which cause not only aches and pain, but also fatigue. When you get used to the feeling of stretching out, the process becomes almost meditative and so helps your body literally cool down and let go after working hard. It also improves circulation by allowing blood to flow into tight areas, so you may also feel areas slightly heating up when you stretch.

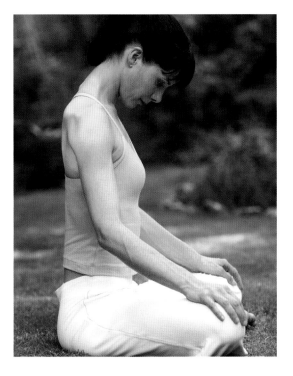

Finally, when doing the Pilates, floor barre and stretch workout, make sure that you always work within your natural range, by which I mean don't do any movement that causes you pain or goes beyond what is comfortable for you. Dancers are naturally more flexible than non-dancers and we can do things with our body that seem easy and normal, but are in fact the direct result of years of training. When you start this programme, you're likely to be less flexible than you think, especially if you haven't exercised for a while and even if you were very flexible as a child. This means you may find that you can't achieve the look in the photographs right away. This is fine because the photographs are here as a guide and more flexibility will come the more you do the programme. For this reason, be sure to take note of the Pilates, floor barre and stretch basics on the following pages and don't overextend your joints or go too fast too soon, because this can lead to injury and won't help you achieve your goals.

As a dancer and mother of two, my ultimate goal is to always take care of my body so that I am in good health and this is essentially what all dancers aim towards. Aside from creating a leaner and stronger body, I've found ballet helps enhance my skills and improves my range of motion in day-to-day life. But to reap these benefits, you need to make sure you do the Pilates, floor barre and stretch workout at least three times a week, as well as stretch your body every day. It sounds a lot, but dancers, no matter how experienced they are, do warm-up barre work every day of their careers. This is not only to keep their muscles in shape, but also to boost their body's physical memory (their body's ability to remember sequences of movement), which will in turn make the workout easier each time you do it.

Try it – I know you won't be sorry.

BEFORE YOU START

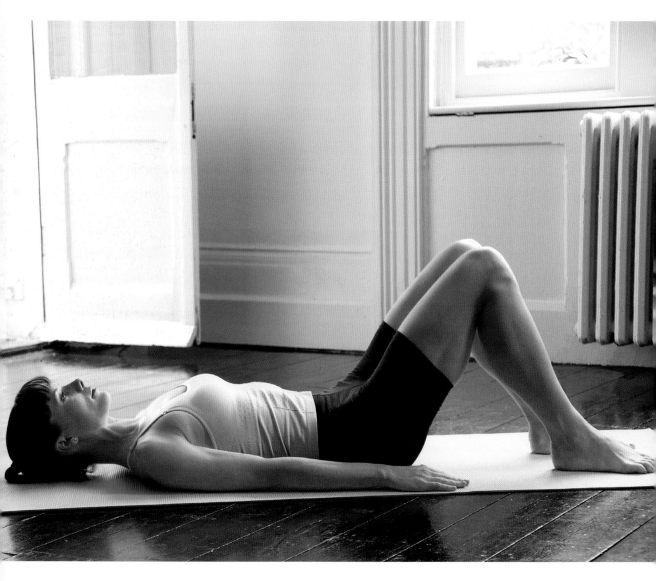

The core basics for Pilates and the floor barre

To gain the most from the Pilates and floor barre workouts, it's important to understand these five elements of the technique.

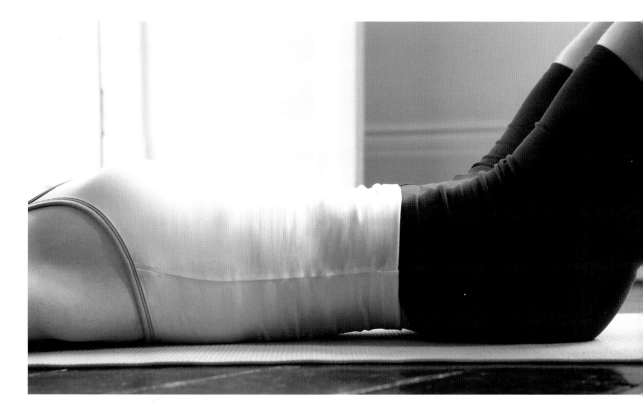

Maintaining your core

Your core is a crucial element of Pilates and the floor barre. To envisage your centre, think of the abdominal and lower back muscles surrounding and supporting your body like a corset. To find your core when lying down, simply pull your bellybutton back towards your spine. Be careful not to pull in so far that you can't breathe and your ribs stick out. The aim is to activate your abdominals so your stomach goes flat, but you can still breathe normally.

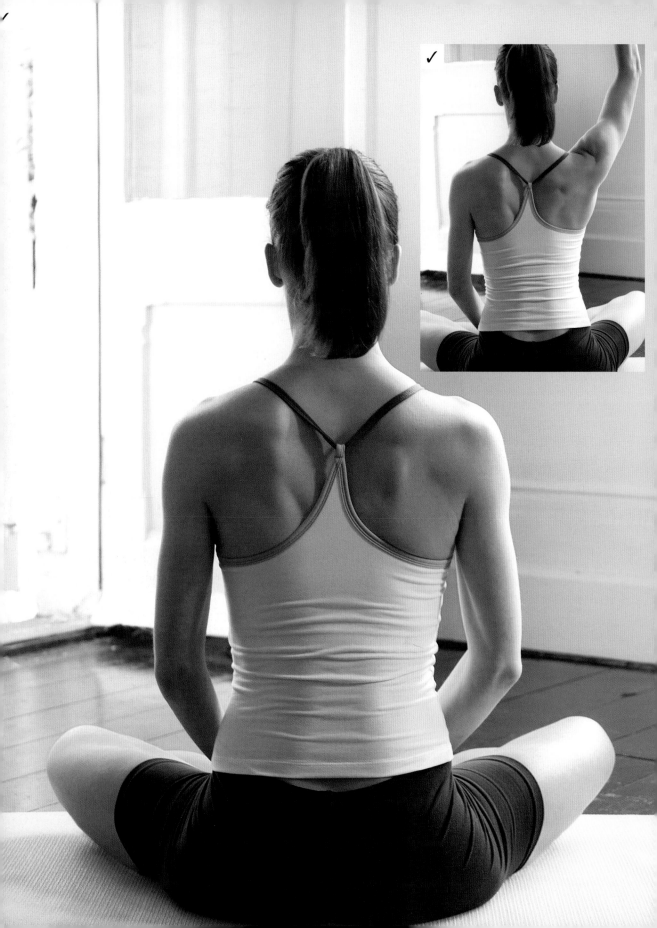

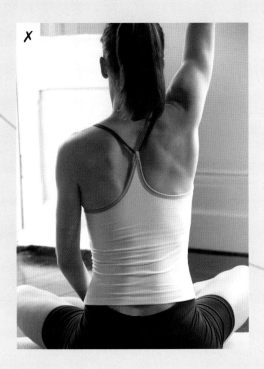

X

Shoulder stabilization

Most of us walk around with our shoulders hunched up around our ears without even realizing they are raised. What this means is that for most of the day, our shoulders are lifted and held in position rather than kept in a relaxed state. Many people also suffer from sore shoulders and neck pain because they don't hold their shoulder blades stable when they lift and raise their arms. To mobilize the shoulders and know where they should be when doing the Pilates warm up and the floor barre exercises, lift both your shoulders up to your ears and roll them backwards (breathing normally as you do this). Imagine a space between your shoulder blades and allow them to slide down your spine (this supports your arms as you lift them). This is where your shoulders should be when starting an exercise: stabilized yet relaxed.

Keeping a relaxed upper body

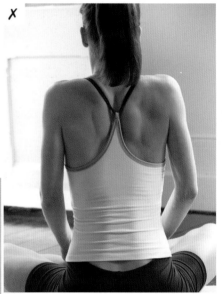

In ballet, and therefore in this programme, the upper body remains relaxed at all times (take a look at any of the dancers in a ballet production to see this). To do this, keep your shoulders stable and your ribs dropped. There should never be a ledge above your waist where your ribs start; your ribs should be in a smooth line with your stomach.

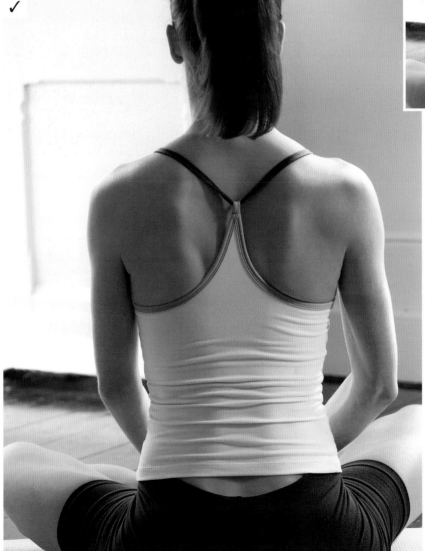

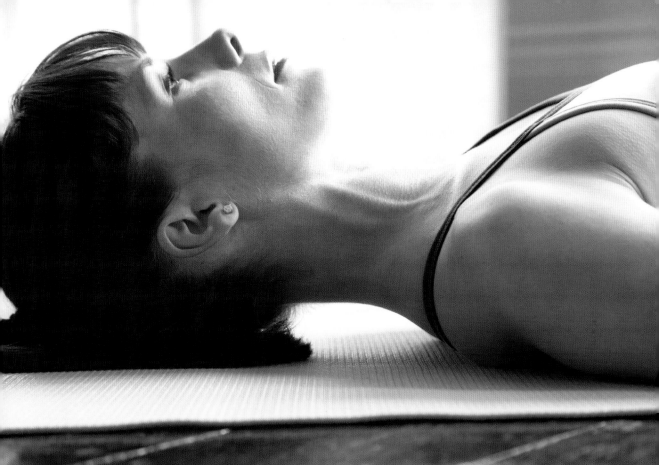

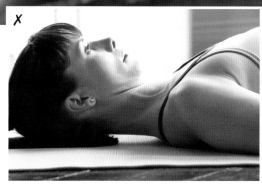

X

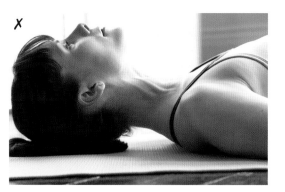

X

The lengthening of the neck

The right neck position is also essential in Pilates and the floor barre to help avoid injury. Whether you're lying, standing or sitting, always imagine your chin moving back closer to your neck and the crown of your head being pulled upwards by a string (do it right and your body will automatically move into a strong postural position). If you can't find this position lying down, place a small rolled-up hand towel under your neck.

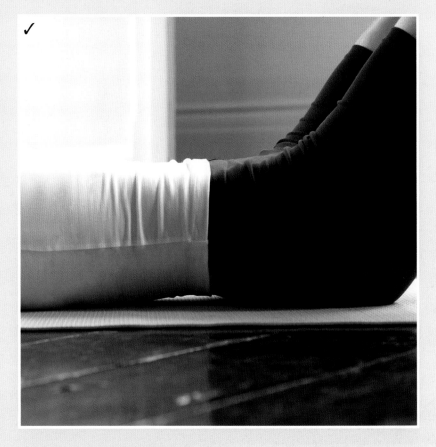

Neutral spine

When lying on your back, the spine should never be pressed flat against the floor. There should always be a natural curve to your lower back. This is a neutral spine and it's the ideal position for your back during the Pilates and floor barre exercises because it places the least amount of stress on your spine.

- To find the correct position, lie down on the floor on your back with your knees bent at a ninety-degree angle, feet parallel and hip-width apart.

- Allow a natural small curve to form at your lower back. Do not press your back into the floor or arch your back the opposite way.

- When you are in 'neutral' your tailbone should be dropped into the floor and you should be able to easily slide a flat hand under your waist.

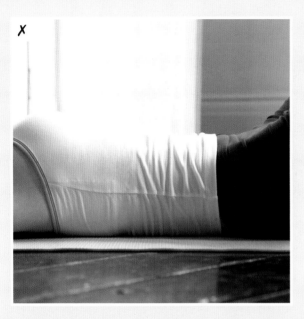

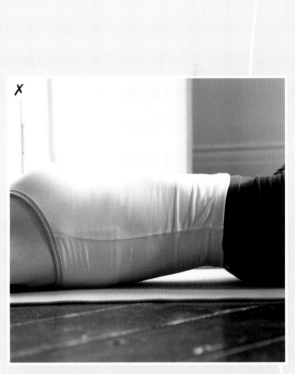

When lying on your back, the spine should never be pressed flat against the floor, or become too arched.

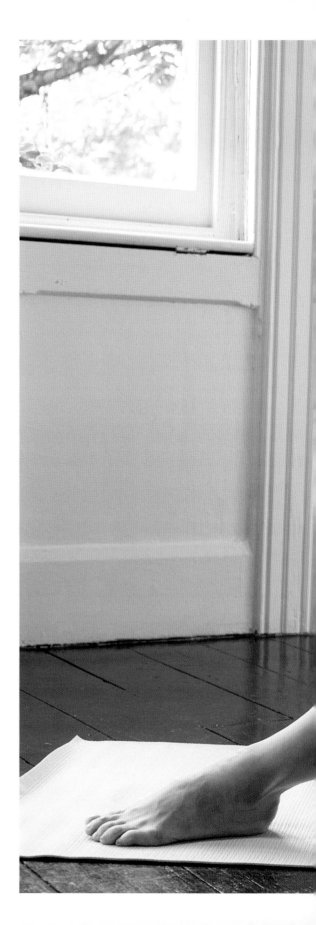

What you need to start

- Enough floor space so that you can stretch out fully

- A wall, preferably with no skirting (for the floor barre)

- A mat (optional)

- A small hand towel that you can roll up and place under your neck

- Clothing that allows for movement

Basic rules

- Keep your stomach muscles engaged at all times when doing both the Pilates and floor barre workouts. This will support your back and make it easier to do the movements

- Warm up and cool down every time you do the programme

- Choose the same time of day, three times a week, to ensure that you get into a routine

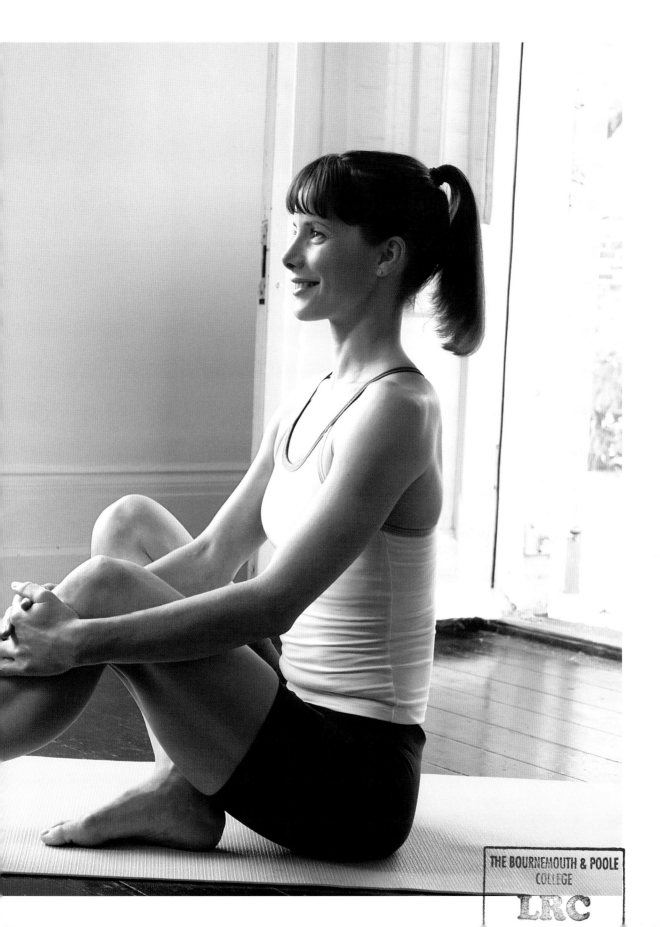

Music

All dancers are inspired by music. It's just impossible for us not to be, and for me, music in all its various forms is one of the most wonderful things about dancing. Apart from the fact that it would be impossible to imagine ballet without music (though it's been done in modern ballet), music is vital to the choreography of dance because it helps lead us through the movements and dictates our pace. In fact it's so important that when we are learning a new dance piece, we often get the music a few weeks ahead of time so we can listen to it over and over for inspiration and get used to the changes and tempo.

It's for this reason that music can be used throughout this floor barre and why you may find it incredibly helpful, not to mention encouraging, while you exercise. In my experience, not only will the right kind of music encourage you to improve on every move, but the accent, rhythm and phrasing of the music will also help you to stay in count and find your extension and stretch.

With regards to what music to listen to while you exercise, the choice is yours. Below are just a few of my favourite classical pieces that I've chosen not only because they work well with the floor barre and Pilates workout, but also because I feel classical music has the right tempo for barre work. Of course, music is incredibly personal so do listen to a selection of music first and see what you can find a rhythm in and what doesn't grate on you and make you feel tense, and then choose accordingly.

Whatever you select, remember to opt for something you feel comfortable with as well as something that enhances, and doesn't take over and distract you from, the exercises. At the same time, pay attention to how you're feeling because, depending on your day's temperament, you may need to hear something more relaxing or invigorating to help you through the workout.

Of all the classical music out there, music written especially for the ballet is perhaps the most natural choice for the floor barre. It's inspiring and easy to move to because the composer naturally took dancing into account while composing it. However, if you're going to do this workout three times a week, I'd also suggest you do experiment and see what suits you best. That way you won't get bored and you can figure out what suits your floor barre style best.

Personally, I love listening and dancing to dramatic-sounding music. On the classical side, Mozart's Requiem and Fauré's Requiem, and on the contemporary side, Jamiroquai and Lenny Kravitz. For me, music is something I like to experiment with so I can see how different pieces make me feel, though I suspect I will always love classical music because I find it simple and clear as well as strong and fluid. What's more, if you've got children I've found you can't go wrong with a classical sound. I played it to my children when I was pregnant and found that it then really helped soothe them when they were unsettled after they were born. Even now, I play it on long car journeys because I find that it helps calm things down.

So whether you're a classical fan or not, do try to give lots of different types of composers a try. Challenge yourself to listen to diverse pieces so that you can find something that not only inspires and energizes you but also encourages you to get the most out of the floor barre and standing programme.

Darcey's classical choices

- Pavane Op. 50, by Gabriel Fauré

- Piano Concerto No. 2 in F Op. 102–II, by
  Dmitri Shostakovich

- Gymnopédie No. 1, by Erik Satie

- Nocturne in E Flat Major Op. 9/2, by Frédéric Chopin

- Meditation (Thaïs, Act 2 Scene 1), by Jules Massenet

- Clarinet Concerto in A, K. 622, Wolfgang Amadeus Mozart

- Piano Concerto No. 21 in C ('Elvira Madigan'),
  K. 467 – II: Andante, by Wolfgang Amadeus Mozart

- Clair de Lune, by Claude Debussy

- Trumpet Concerto in D Minor, by Benedetto Marcello

The Workout

THE PILATES WARM UP

While it's always tempting to skip a warm up, don't do it. Warming up properly is essential for everyone, not just dancers, because not only does a good warm up allow your muscles to stretch, but it also prepares your body for a longer workout. In ballet, it's essential to protect your body from injury any way you can, so a good warm up is always essential.

The joy of this Pilates warm up is that you can do it alone when you're time-starved and it will still help you improve your flexibility and mobility, as well as improve your technique in the floor barre. The exercises here have been designed to be completed in twenty minutes, but as the key is to always do what feels like natural stretches for you (meaning you shouldn't force your body into positions that feel painful or too uncomfortable), it may take longer at first.

Also bear in mind, as with ballet, every move in Pilates has a purpose. To skip a step or exercise because it seems easy or unimportant, or not to take an exercise to its full range of movement, will not only shorten your muscles, but also negate the benefit of the technique itself. So although Pilates may seem slow and methodical to start with, or not as exciting as the ballet moves, after you have mastered the basics, you'll quickly see how it is a dynamic and highly effective way to build a long and lean body fast.

Pelvic floor muscles

Step one: Lie on the floor on your back with your legs bent at a ninety-degree angle and feet hip-width apart. Place your arms by your sides. Now, imagine you are about to pee and then stop – these are your pelvic floor muscles.

Step two: Squeeze these muscles by pulling them upwards to your stomach. Hold for four counts and release.

Repeat ten times.

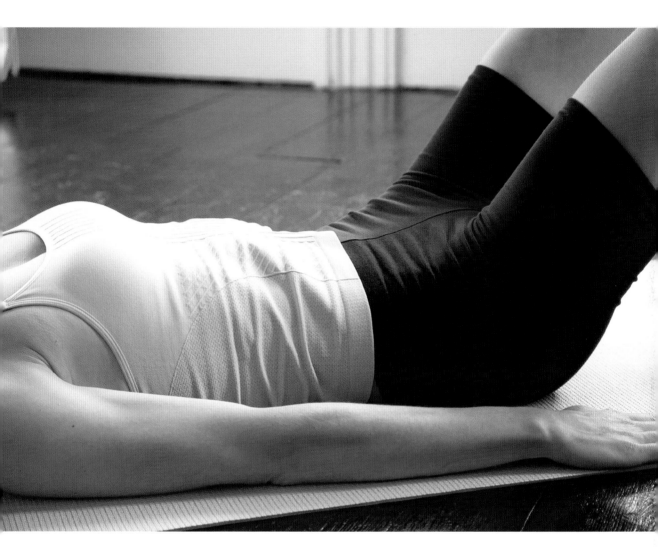

Key Point:	Helps you connect with your centre
Works:	Your pelvic floor

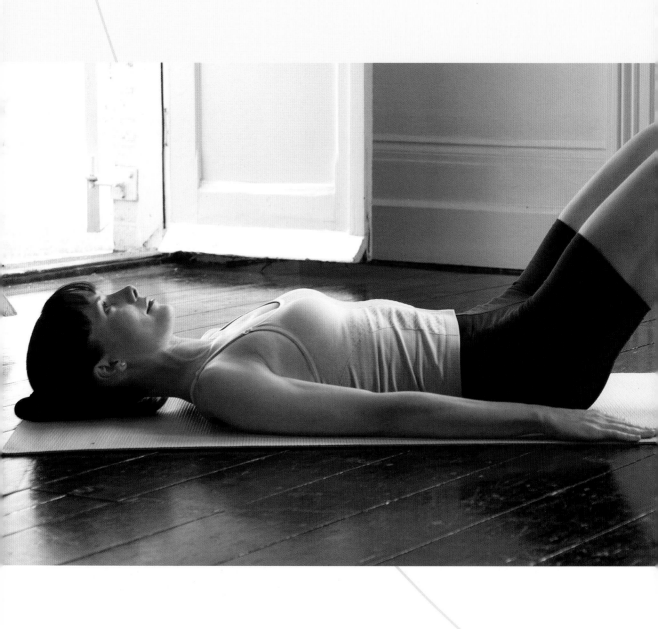

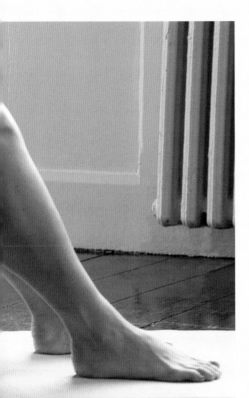

Single leg raise

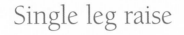

Step one: Lie on the floor with your legs bent at a ninety-degree angle, feet parallel and hip-width apart. Place your arms by your sides and pull your bellybutton to your spine to engage your stomach muscles.

Step two: Slowly inhale and at the same time let one leg float upwards off the floor, bringing the knee over the hip and keeping your leg at a ninety-degree angle. Hold for two counts and, on the exhale, return the leg to the floor in two counts.

Step three: Repeat with the other leg.

Repeat five times on each leg, alternating between them.

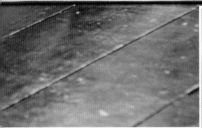

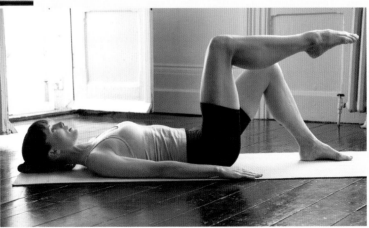

Works: | Your abdominals

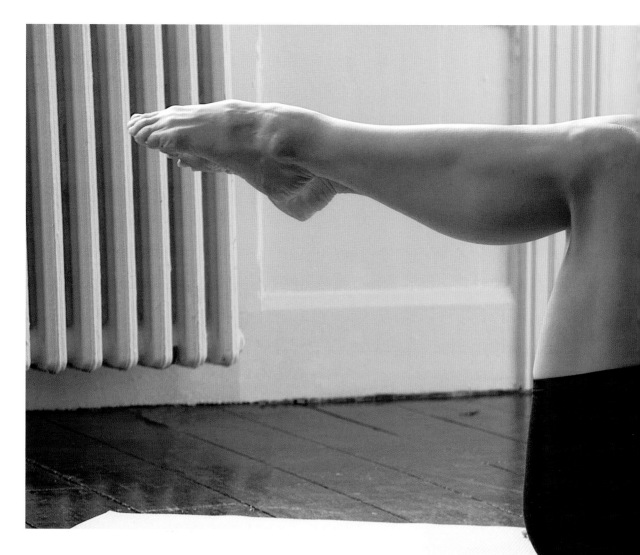

Double leg raise

Step one: Lie on the floor with your legs bent at a ninety-degree angle, feet parallel and hip-width apart. Place your arms by your sides.

Step two: As you inhale, slowly pull your stomach muscles in and let one leg float up until the knee is over the hip, keeping your leg at a ninety-degree angle. Then bring your other leg up to the same position and hold for two counts.

Step three: Exhale and allow the first leg to go back down in two counts, and then the other. Control your legs on the way down to the floor with your stomach muscles.

Repeat ten times.

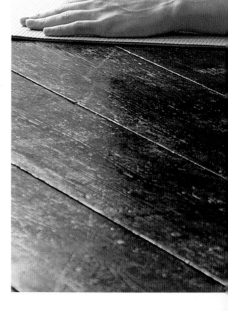

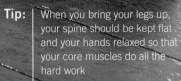

Tip: When you bring your legs up, your spine should be kept flat and your hands relaxed so that your core muscles do all the hard work

Works: Your abdominals and hamstrings

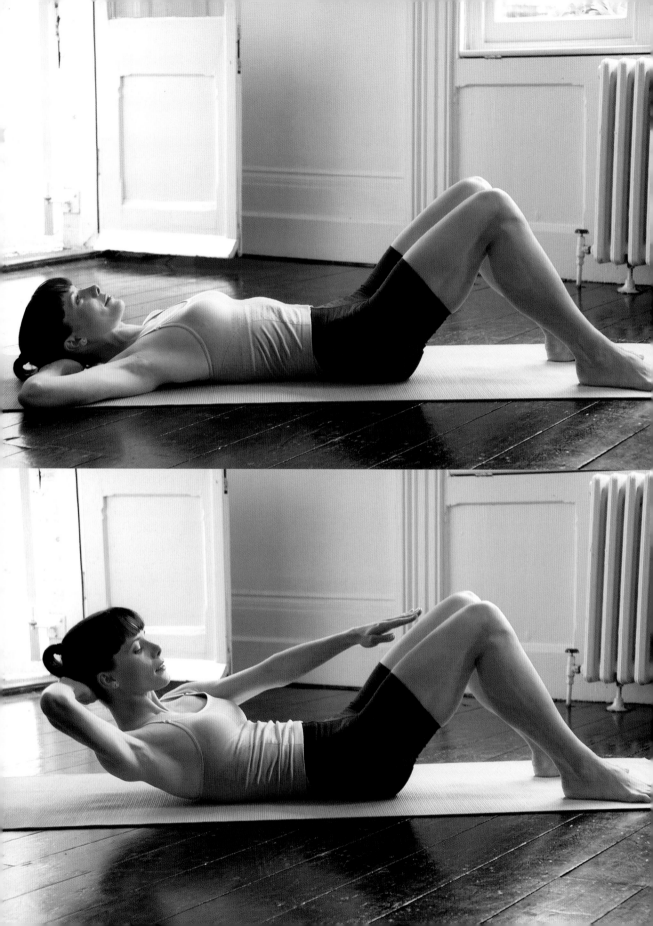

Tip:	If this exercise is too hard, keep both arms behind your head and as you curl forwards, twist the elbow of one arm towards the opposing knee. Curl back and repeat on the other side
Works:	Your side muscles
Key point:	Works on whittling your waist down

Obliques

Step one: Lie on the floor with your knees bent, feet parallel and hip-width apart. Place one hand behind your head and the other by your side. Inhale.

Step two: On the exhale, scoop in your abdominals and curl your head and chest off the floor (keep your gaze on your knees and don't pull your head forward from the neck). Twist your body and move your free arm to your opposing knee.

Step three: Exhale and curl back to the floor.

Repeat five times on each side.

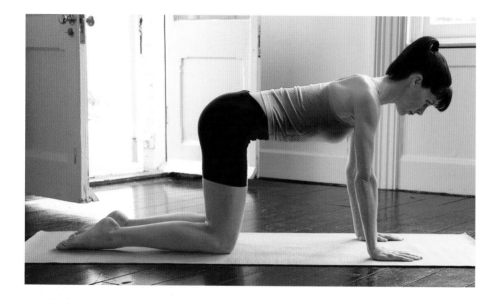

Dog

Step one: Face the floor on all fours. Knees should be under hips, arms under your shoulders and head aligned with your spine in a straight line.

Step two: Breathing normally and maintaining a flat back, lift one leg off the floor, keeping it bent at a ninety-degree angle. Bring it in line with your hip and then return to the starting position.

Repeat five times on each leg.

Tip: | Pull your stomach in to keep your back straight and draw your shoulder blades down to stop your shoulders hunching up

Works: | Your hamstrings, glutes and abdominals

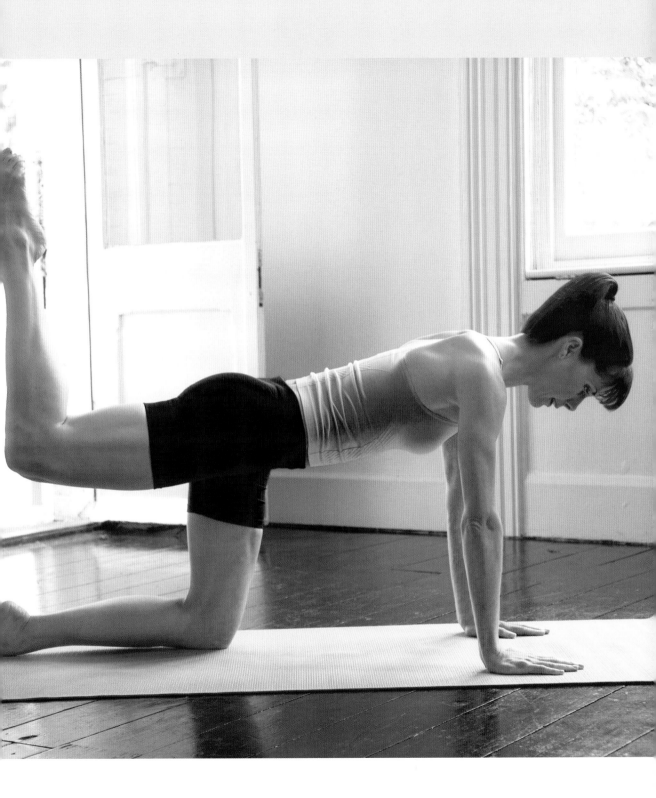

Opposite arm and leg

Step one: Get on to all fours on the floor. Knees should be under hips, arms under your shoulders and head aligned with your spine in a straight line. Keep your shoulders pulled down.

Works: | Your hamstrings and abdominals

Step two: Inhale and, pulling in your stomach muscles to support you, stretch out one arm and the opposing leg at the same time. Bring your arm in line with your shoulder, your leg in line with your hip and reach through the fingers and toes.

Step three: Exhale and return to the starting position. Repeat with the other arm and leg.

Repeat five times on each leg, alternating between them.

Sphinx into a roll up

Step one: Face the floor on all fours and, without moving your hands, draw your bottom back to sit on your heels. Extend your hands along the floor in front of you as far as they will go (think of a sphinx). Your bottom should now be on your heels and your forehead on the floor.

Step two: From this position inhale and, drawing your navel to your spine, slowly roll upwards one vertebra at a time to come up to a kneeling position. Keep your bottom on your heels and let your arms drop to your sides.

Step three: Exhale and roll back down to the starting position

Repeat five times.

1

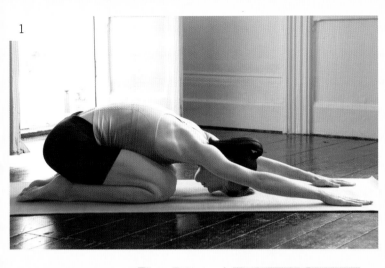

2i

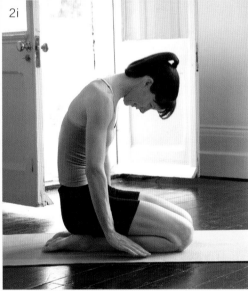

2ii

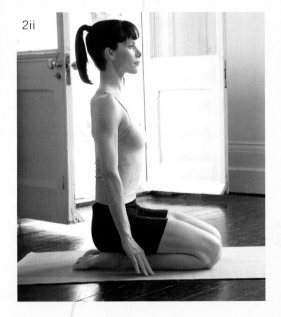

Works: | Your spine, abdominals and neck

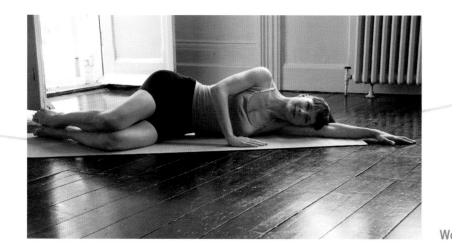

Tip: Don't turn your hip out as you move your knee

Works: Your glutes

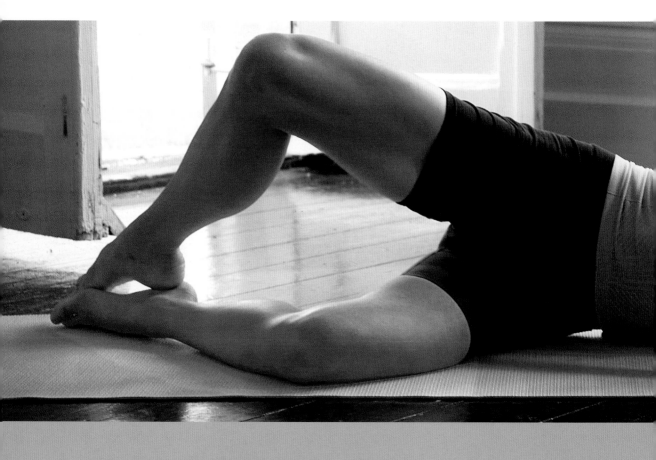

Clams (I)

Step one: Lie on one side with your knees bent in front of you, feet together (soles in line with your back) and your stomach pulled in. Keep your lower arm extended under your head and your other hand on the floor in front of you for support.

Step two: Inhale and on the exhale, keeping your feet together and bottom taut, lift your top knee so it points towards the ceiling (think of the knees opening like a clam shell). Make sure you don't sink into your waist.

Step three: Inhale and return to the starting position.

Repeat ten times on each leg.

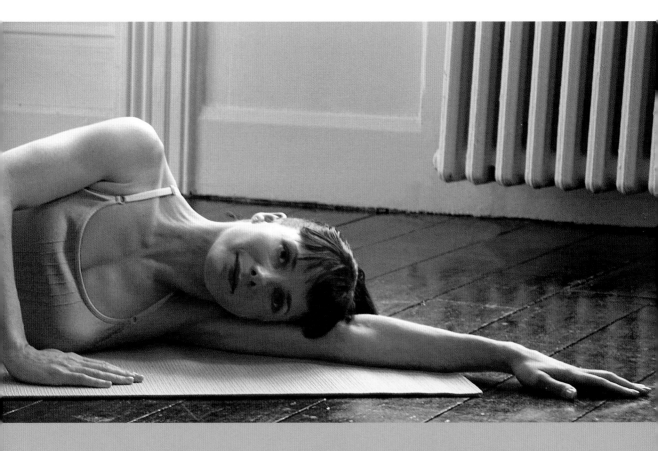

Clams (II)

Step one: Lie on one side with your knees bent in front of you, feet together (soles in line with your back) and your stomach pulled in. Keep your lower arm extended under your head and your other hand on the floor in front of you for support.

Step two: Inhale and on the exhale, making sure you don't sink into your waist, lift your top knee so it's pointing towards the ceiling. Keeping your leg in this position, lift it towards your hip.

Step three: Breathe normally and lower your leg until your feet are touching.

Repeat ten times on each leg.

Works: | Your glutes

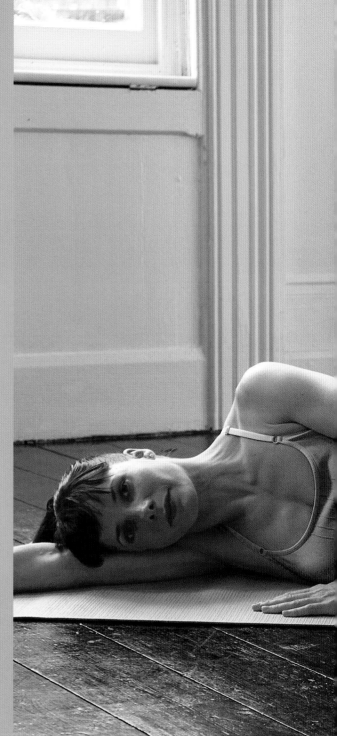

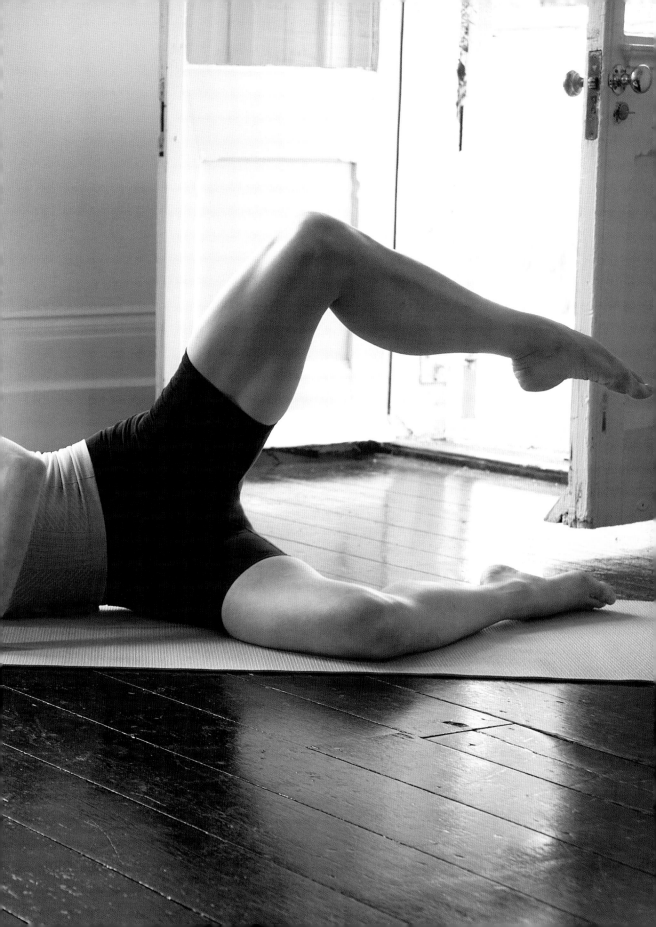

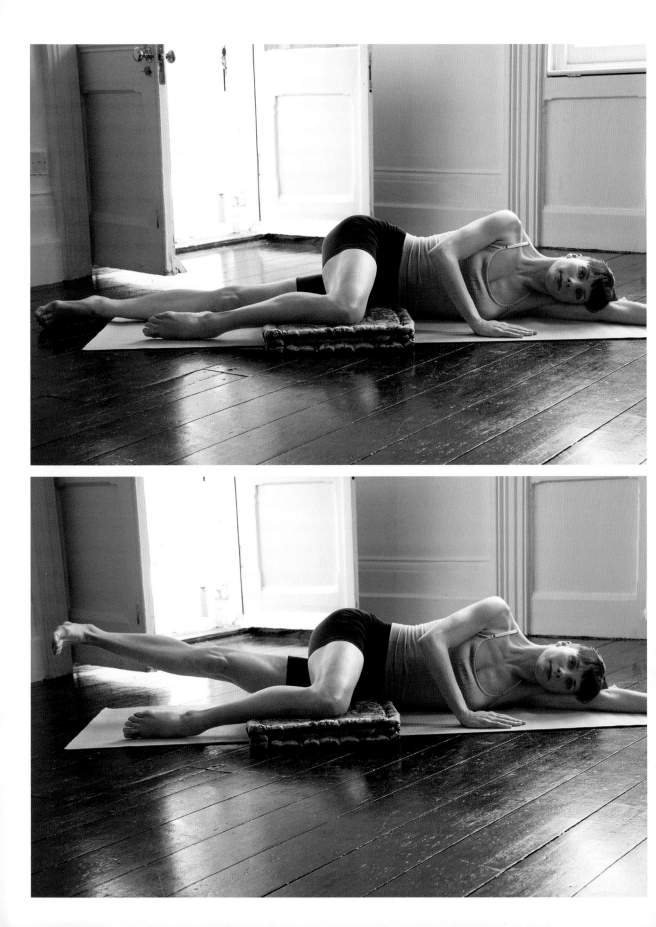

Tip:	To lengthen your leg when lifting, push through the heel
Works:	Your inside thighs

Inside thigh lifts

Step one: Lie on one side and put your upper leg and knee on a cushion in front of your body, keeping your lower leg extended underneath. Don't let your hip roll forward: it should remain level with your spine. Keep one arm extended under your head and the other in front of you for support.

Step two: Breathing normally, flex the foot of the lower leg and lift and lengthen it away from the floor. Hold for ten counts.

Turn over and repeat on the opposing leg.

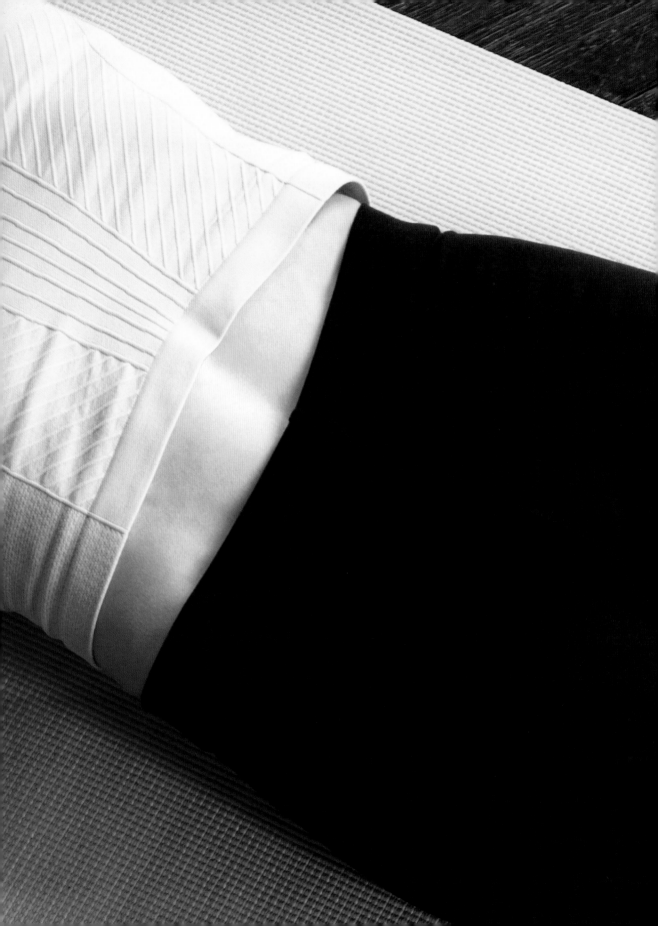

This exercise creates flexibility in an area where muscles can become quite tight.

Hip hitching

Step one: Lie on the floor on your back with your legs straight and feet hip-width apart. Have your arms by your sides and your stomach pulled in. Keep your ribs dropped and upper body relaxed.

Step two: Keeping your bottom on the floor, hitch one hip up and at the same time stretch out the opposing leg (imagine your leg pulling away from your hip joint).

Do five hitches on each side.

Tip: The legs work in opposition here, so as one leg hitches up, the other lengthens

Works: Your hip flexors (the group of muscles passing through the pelvis that act to flex the hips and rotate the lower spine)

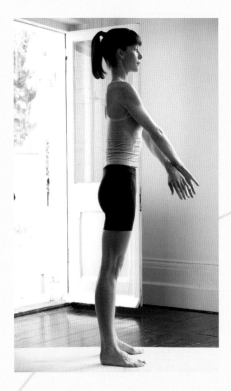

Figures of eight

Step one: Stand square-on in front of a mirror with your feet hip-width apart and knees slightly bent, arms by your sides and stomach pulled in.

Step two: Inhale and, keeping your arms straight, cross them in front of you, palms facing each other but not touching. Now turn your arms out so that your palms are facing the ceiling. Keeping your shoulders down, swing both arms outwards and behind you as far as they will go.

Step three: Now turn your arms in so your palms are facing backwards, and then swing them back to the starting position.

Repeat ten times.

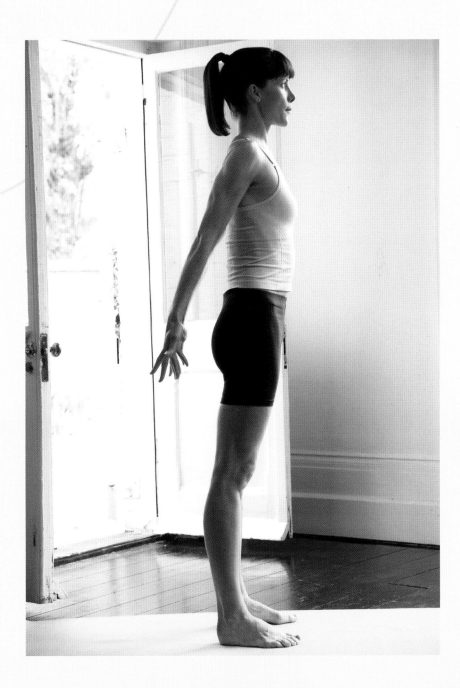

Tip: | Imagine each arm makes a large figure of eight.
Make the whole movement continuous and flowing

Works: | Your triceps (underarm muscles)

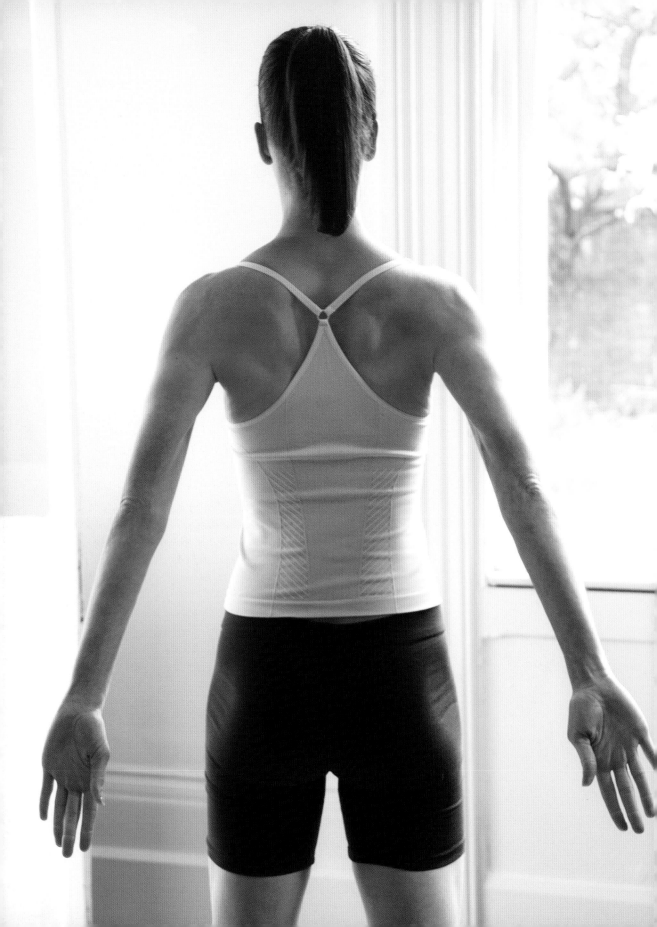

Tip:	Remember to breathe normally as you do this
Works:	Your triceps

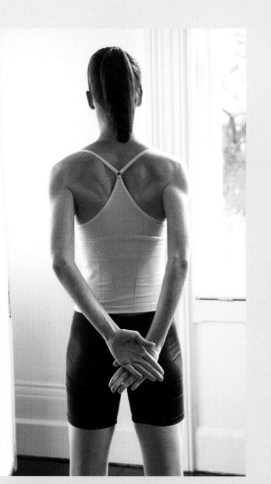

Beating hundreds
(derrière)

Step one: Stand with your feet hip-width apart and your legs slightly bent, your shoulders pulled down and your stomach pulled in. Have your arms by your sides with palms facing backwards.

Step two: Keeping your arms straight, push them back as far as they will go. From this position, cross your arms behind you, swing them back out, and then cross them behind you again. As you cross palms behind you, you should alternate which one is on top.

Continue this action in a controlled movement. Aim to do a hundred beats.

Cat and reverse cat (spine stretch)

Step one: Get on to all fours. Your knees should be under your hips and arms under your shoulders. Make sure your head is aligned with your spine and your stomach is pulled in.

Step two: Inhale and push your spine upwards so that your upper body curls (imagine a cat's back curling). Relax your neck and let your head drop.

Step three: From this position, exhale, drop your bellybutton towards the floor, and then lift your breastbone and head towards the ceiling.

Repeat this sequence five times.

Works: Your back, neck and shoulder muscles

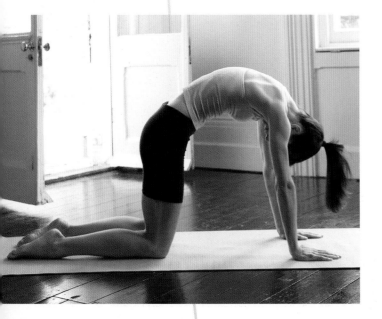

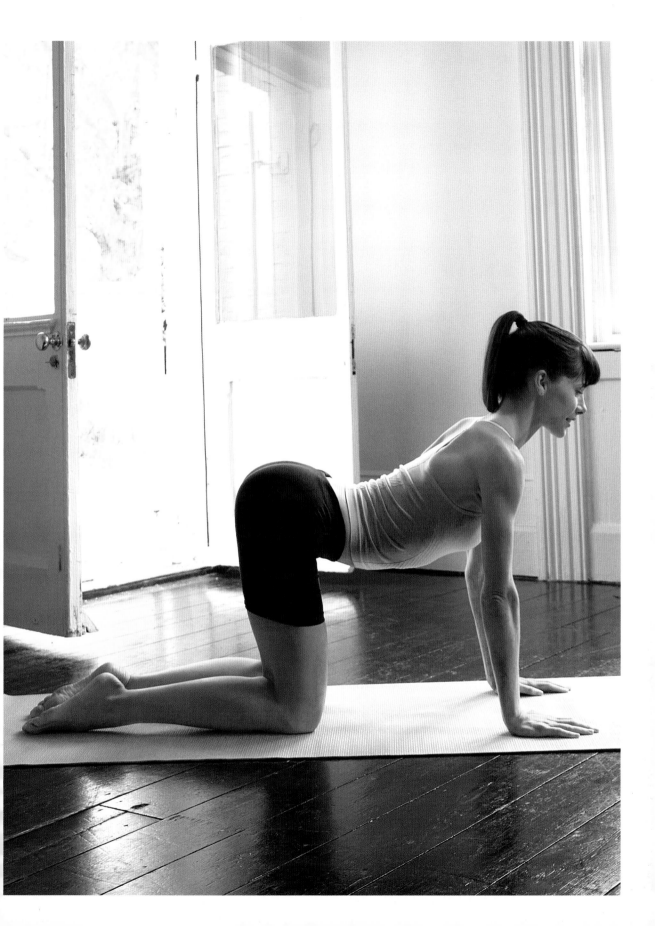

THE FLOOR BARRE

Now that you've finished the Pilates warm up, you're ready to begin the main part of my unique workout: the floor barre programme which I have adapted for people who have never tried a dance class. The floor barre is designed to give you a feel for how dancers exercise at the barre and so is a very precise and technical type of exercise that has great benefits for the body. As barre work is really where the training and forming of muscles occur for dancers, to get the most out of it always focus on your technique and making your movements as precise and as controlled as possible.

Also, remember that each exercise is there for a reason. The *pliés* (knee bends) are for the hips, the *tendu* (a brushing movement of the foot) helps warm up the ankles, and the *dégagé* (a brushing movement in which the foot comes off the floor at a forty-five-degree angle) helps increase the speed of your movements. The *rond de jambe* (a semicircle drawn by the foot) helps to increase the leg's turnout and *frappés* (a striking movement with the foot) will help quicken your reflexes. The *adagio* (a slow movement) and *fondu* (a one-legged knee bend) both increase suppleness and control, while *grand battements* (high throwing kicks) increase strength and stamina.

Like Pilates, the basis of the floor barre is a strong core. Firm abdominal muscles will not only support your front and back (by acting like a corset around the body), but also help you to move and take the pressure off your lower back. If you suffer from lower back pain, you'll very likely have weak stomach muscles. This is why it's important to maintain your core at all times during the floor barre. Pull your navel back towards your spine to activate your abdominals so that your stomach goes flat, but you can still breathe normally and execute movements.

All the exercises here are progressive (in the same way that ballet is), which means each exercise gives you the strength, balance and technique to prepare you for the next step. Moves are also repeated in various sequences so they slowly warm up the muscles and stick in your mind. So again, don't skip parts or rush through the exercises that you find easier. The more you follow the floor barre and make it part of your workout, the easier the exercises will be to follow, the faster your muscles will react and you'll see amazing results for your body. It will also give you a flavour of what a dancer's barre can be like.

The essential floor barre basics

Turnout

Before beginning any ballet exercises, all dancers must find the correct placement at the barre and this is the same for the floor barre. Before starting, always turn out your legs (this is what the rotation of the legs is known as in the ballet world). To do this:

Step one: Lie on the floor with your legs straight, pull your navel gently to your spine and keep your upper body relaxed.

Step two: Now rotate both legs outwards, starting the movement from the tops of your thighs. To help yourself, imagine the very tops of your thighs wrapping around your bottom. If you do this correctly, your hips will open outwards and your feet will move to first position: heels touching, toes pointing outwards.

Step three: Lie in this position for thirty seconds to get used to the feeling.

The supporting leg

In floor barre and barre work, all movement starts with your right leg. The supporting leg is known as the 'root' and must stay still and turned out during each exercise. This keeps the opposing hip turned out and acts as a support for the moving leg.

Pointing your foot

We all imagine we can point our foot perfectly, but in ballet a perfectly pointed foot is straight and long with toes that don't curl or kink at the end. This is the most strengthening position for the entire foot. To get this right:

Step one: Sit against a wall with your legs straight in front of you.

Step two: Flex your feet so your calves stretch and your toes point towards the ceiling (known as bad toes).

Step three: Now, keeping your toes relaxed, bend your ankles and point your toes without curling them (known as good toes). Imagine you are creating a straight line with your foot. This is a pointed foot.

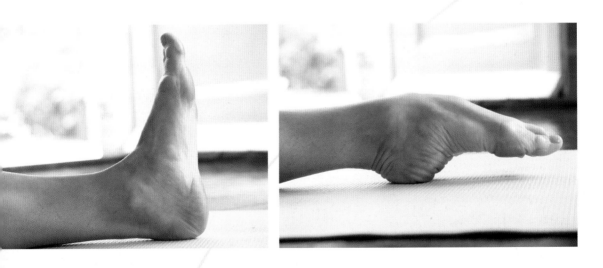

The five positions of the legs and arms lying down

The positions of the arms should be done in a soft, fluid and continuous movement rather than fast and jerky.

first position

1

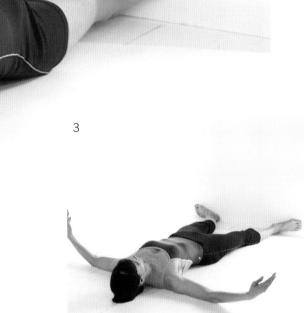

3

Prepare

Legs: Lie on the floor with your feet touching a wall. Keeping your heels together, turn your legs out from the hip. Your feet should be flexed and toes pointed outwards.

Arms: Keeping your shoulders and upper body relaxed, your arms should be long and slightly curved into a long oval shape with palms facing down and resting on your hips just below your pelvis. Your elbows should be lifted off the floor.

First position

Legs: First position for the legs is the same as prepare position, with heels together, legs turned out from the hips, feet flexed and toes pointed outwards.

Arms: From prepare position, bring your arms to bellybutton height in front of your body, keeping them long and slightly curved and your palms facing your navel. Imagine you are hugging a large beach ball.

Second position

Legs: Starting in first position (left), slide both feet out along the wall to the sides until your heels are just over hip-width apart. Weight should be distributed evenly between both legs. Legs should be turned out, feet flexed and toes pointed outwards.

Arms: Reaching through your fingers open your arms to the side of your body, just below shoulder height. There should be a slight curve in your arms and your palms should face upwards. The top part of the arms should rest lightly on the floor.

Third position

Legs: From second position, slide both feet back to first position and place your right foot in front of your left foot with your right heel touching the middle of your left foot below the toe joint. Legs should be straight and turned out, feet flexed and toes pointed outwards. This can be hard the first time.

Arms: There is no third position when lying down. Go back to prepare position.

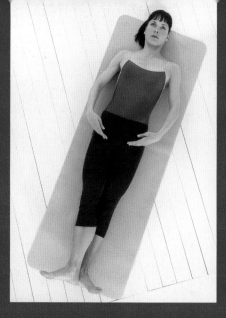

Fourth position

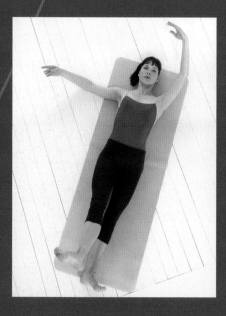

Legs: From third position, raise your right foot upwards so that it's placed in front of the left foot about a step away. Keep your legs straight and turned out, feet flexed and toes pointed outwards, and support yourself from your stomach.

Arms: From prepare position, first lift your arms to first position, then raise your left arm over your head so that the palm is facing your forehead and still in sight without you having to move your head. Open your right arm out to second position. Keep both arms slightly curved.

Fifth position

Legs: From fourth position, lower your right foot so that your heel is against your left big toe. Your right knee should be over your left knee, legs straight and turned out, feet flexed and toes pointed outwards. This position is difficult to do lying down; standing up it's easier to turn your legs outwards because the weight of your body helps you. Just do the best you can and don't force your legs into the position.

Arms: From fourth position, raise your right arm above your head so that both palms are facing your forehead. Your arms should be slightly curved. In fifth position, you should still be able to see your hands without moving your head.

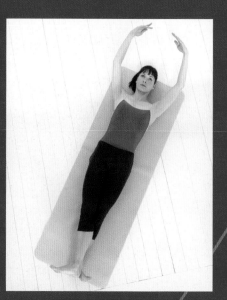

Basic rules

- With the floor barre exercises, inhale to start the movement and exhale on the effort, but breathe normally throughout

- The starting position for all floor barre exercises is lying on your back with your legs straight and turned out, feet in first position, stomach muscles engaged and arms in second position (see page 78)

- Familiarize yourself with the ballet positions on the previous pages by practising each one six times

- With floor barre exercises, work always begins with the right foot

- Familiarize yourself with the following ballet terminology before you start the floor barre:

  - o *Demi-plié* (a half knee bend)

  - o *Grand plié* (a deep knee bend)

  - o *Tendu* (a brushing movement of the foot either in front (*devant*) or to the side (*à la seconde*)

  - o *Glissé* (a sliding movement of the foot in which it comes off the floor)

  - o *Relevé* (a rise to the balls of the feet)

  - o *Cou-de-pied* (a ballet position in which one foot is placed in front of the opposing ankle)

  - o *Fondu* (a one-legged knee bend)

  - o *Rond de jambe* (a semicircle drawn by the foot either on the floor (à terre) or in the air (*en l'air*)

  - o *Frappé* (a striking movement with the foot)

  - o *Adagio* (a slow movement)

  - o *Grand battement* (a high throwing kick)

  - o *Port de bras* (a movement of the arms from one position to another)

Warm up (I)

Step one: Sit upright on the floor with your knees bent and feet parallel in front of you. Sit up out of your hips and let your arms support you at the sides of your body. Pull your navel to your spine to support your back and think of the top of your head reaching towards the ceiling. Breathe in.

Step two: Breathe out, take your arms off the floor and raise them to first position (arms in front of you, palms at bellybutton height and facing inwards). Keep your shoulders pulled down, your upper body relaxed and your arms slightly curved. Breathe in.

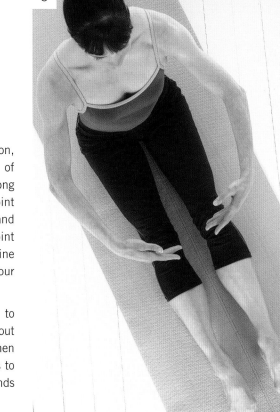

Step three: Breathe out and from this position, remembering to keep sitting up out of your hips, straighten out your legs along the floor. Keeping them parallel, point your feet. Keep your toes relaxed and bend your ankles so your toes point towards the wall in front of you (imagine your feet and toes are an extension of your whole leg pointing in one direction).

Step four: Breathe in and draw your legs back to the starting position. Straighten them out again, point your toes then flex them, then point and flex again. Return your legs to the starting position and place your hands back on the floor by your sides.

Repeat four times.

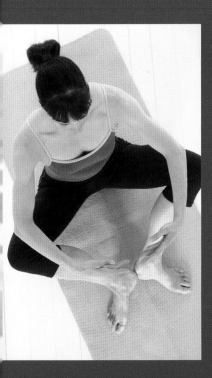

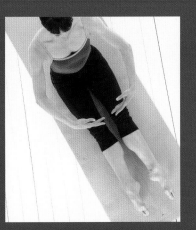

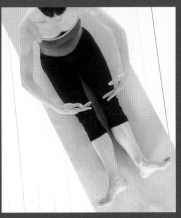

Progression: *Do Warm up (I) following the same process, but starting with knees bent outwards and feet turned out and in first position (heels together, feet flexed and toes pointed outwards). Be sure to keep your feet in this position when straightening your legs and drawing them back in and out again, and then point and flex your toes twice, keeping your feet in first.*

2   3

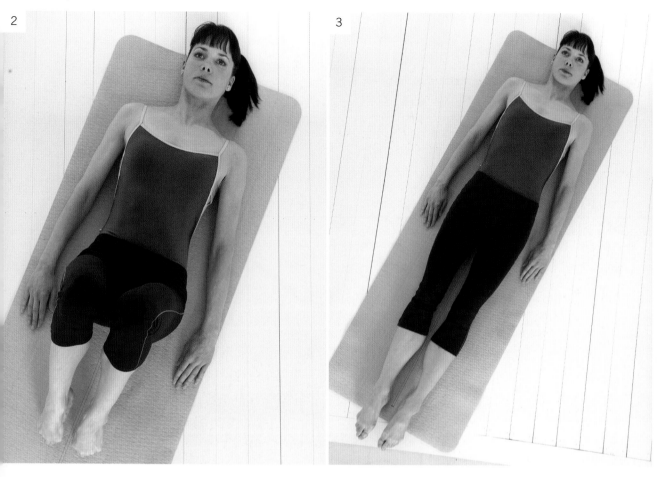

Warm up (II)

Step one: Lie on your back on the floor with your legs straight and parallel and your arms by your sides. Pull your stomach in and relax your upper body. Breathe in. Breathe out. Keep your shoulders pulled down and upper body relaxed. Your arms should be resting by the sides of your body with palms near your hips.

Step two: Breathe in and, bending your knees, brush your feet, with pointed toes, along the floor towards your tailbone as far as they can go.

Step three: Breathe out and let your heels drop to the floor. Slide your legs back along the floor to the starting position. Draw your legs back up to your tailbone and extend them one more time. Then point your toes and flex them, then point and flex again.

Repeat four times.

Progression: Do Warm up (II) following the same process, but starting with legs straight and turned out and feet in first position. When sliding your feet towards your tailbone point them so that at the top of the movement your toes touch. Your knees should point outwards in a froglike shape. Then straighten your legs, moving your feet back to first position, and point and flex your feet twice.

2

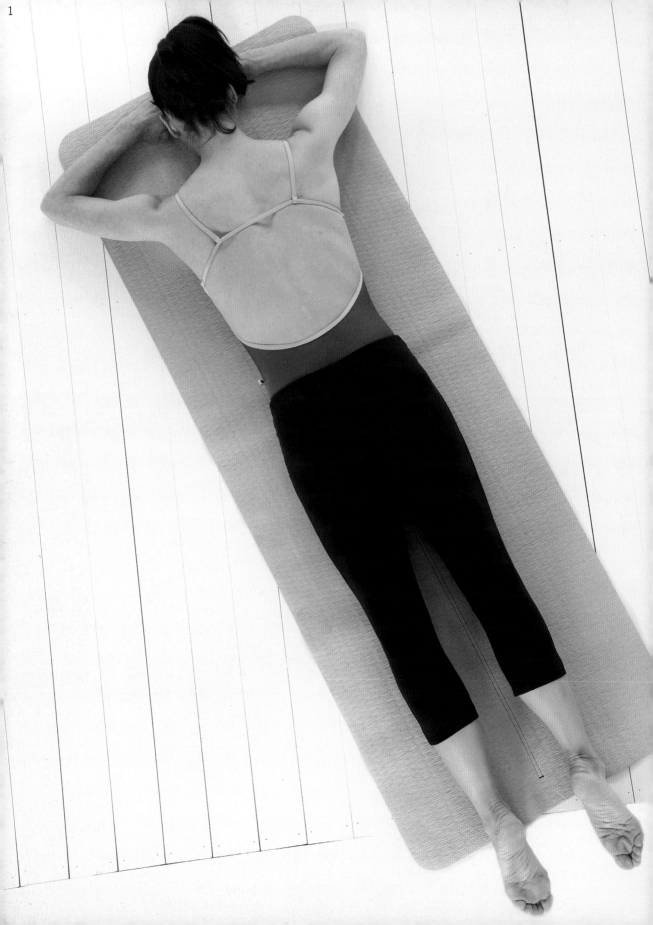

Warm up (III)

Step one: Lie on your front on the floor with your legs straight and parallel and your hands under your forehead. Pull your stomach in and relax your upper body.

Step two: Breathing normally, point your toes and lift your legs to a ninety-degree angle off the floor. Lower your legs back to the floor, flexing your feet as you go. When your toes touch the floor, straighten your legs, lifting your thighs. Relax your legs.

Repeat four times.

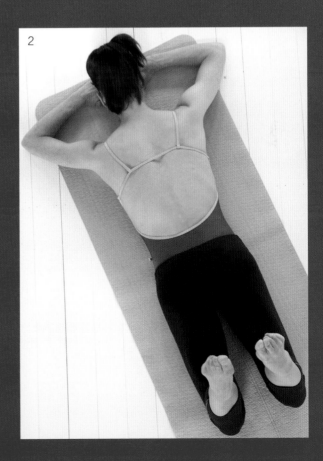

Starting position

This is the starting position
for all floor barre exercises.

Step one: Lie on your back on the floor with your legs straight and turned out from the hip, feet in first position (heels together, feet flexed and toes pointing outwards) and your abdominals held in (think navel to spine).

Step two: Lift your arms to second position by first raising them in front of your body to first position, then, reaching through your fingers, open them out to the sides of your body, just below shoulder height. There should be a slight curve in your arms and your palms should face upwards. You should always move your arms into second position this way.

Tip: If your head is uncomfortable, place a small rolled-up hand towel under your neck

Pliés

Pliés are the basis of everything you do in ballet, so it's important to master them.

Pliés in first
(knee bends in first position)

Step one: In the centre of the room, get into the starting position for the floor barre.

Step two: From this position, do a *demi-plié* (a half knee bend) by bending both your knees and drawing your heels up along the floor halfway towards your tailbone. Think of making a frog shape on the floor with your legs: your knees should stay pointed outwards and your heels should remain in first position as you draw your legs up towards your tailbone.

Step three: Once at the top of the movement, push down through the heels and thighs back to first position.

Count two to draw your feet up and two to extend out. Be sure to keep your stomach muscles engaged throughout the entire exercise. Repeat twice.

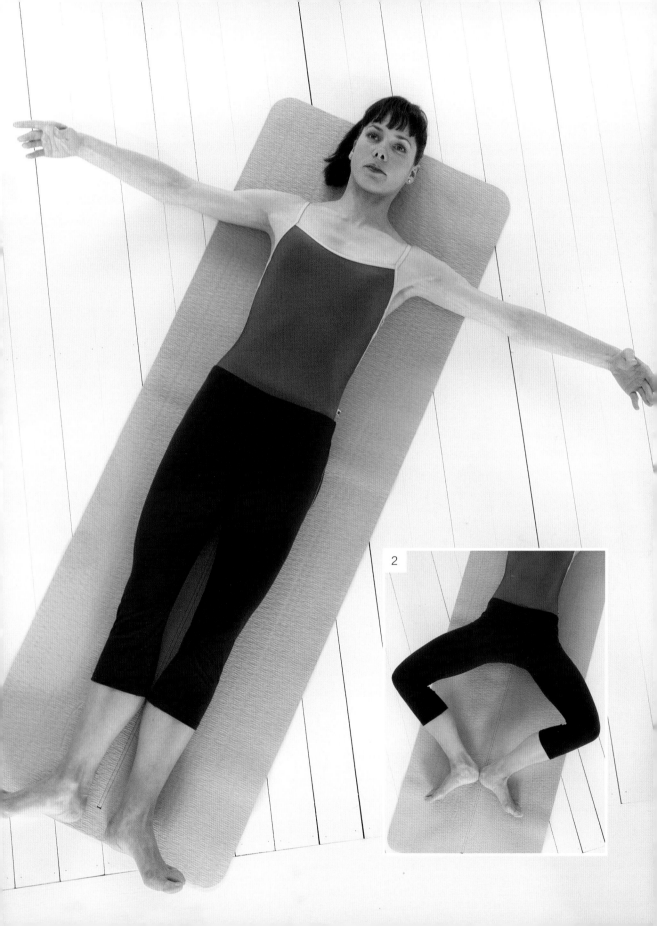

2

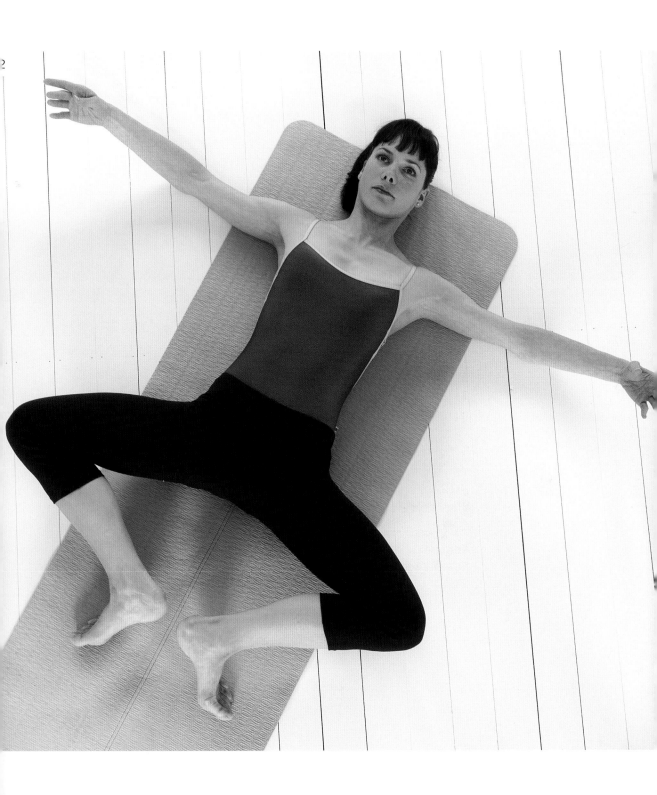

Tip:	To begin with, your knees will not lie flat on the floor. As you progress, however, your hips will open, your inner thighs will relax and your knees will move closer to the floor
Works:	Your inner thighs, abdominals and glutes

Pliés progression
(knee bends progression)

Step one:	Stay in the centre of the room and get into the starting position for the floor barre.
Step two:	This time, do a *grand plié* (a deep knee bend) by bending both your knees and drawing your heels up along the floor as far as they will go. Your knees should stay pointed outwards and your feet should remain in first position.
Step three:	Once at the top of the movement, push down through the heels and thighs back to first position.
	Take four counts to draw in and four counts to extend. Keep your stomach muscles engaged throughout. Repeat twice.

1

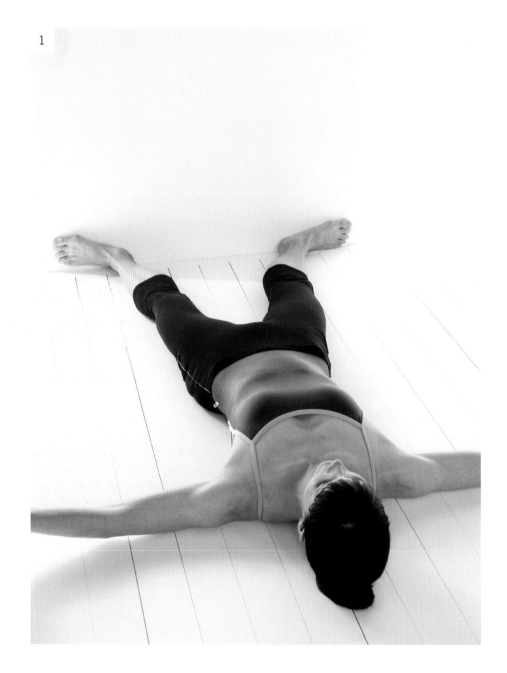

The *plié* is a lot harder in second, and more so on the floor. When dancers do a *plié à la seconde* at the barre, we have our body weight pushing down to help us into position.

Pliés à la seconde (knee bends in second position)

Step one: Move towards a wall and get into the starting position for the floor barre.

Step two: Slide both feet out to second position until your heels are about hip-width apart. Drop your heels so that both feet line up. Your weight should be distributed evenly between both legs and your legs should be turned out.

Step three: In this position, do two *demi-pliés*, keeping your knees pointed outwards and feet in second (think of a starfish shape).

Count four to draw legs in and four to extend back to second position. Repeat twice.

Progression: *From the starting position, slide feet out to second position. Do one* grand plié. *Take four counts to draw legs in and four counts to extend back out to second position. Repeat this sequence twice.*

Tip: Don't take all the tension in your hip flexors (the muscles at the top of your legs that attach your hips to your thighs). Try to consciously relax the tension here and instead use your inside thighs to draw your legs up. Think of a pushing sensation through the heels when extending down

Works: Your inner thighs and opens the hips

Plié relevé (a knee bend followed by a rise to the balls of the feet)

Step one: Stay against the wall and get into the starting position for the floor barre.

Step two: Do a *demi-plié*.

Step three: When your legs return to first position, push on to the balls of your feet. Return your feet to first position where they are flexed. You won't be able to come back to the wall because your body will have naturally moved away when you rose up.

Return to the wall and repeat six times.

2

Warms up:	The feet, ankles and calves
Works:	Your hamstrings, inner thighs and feet

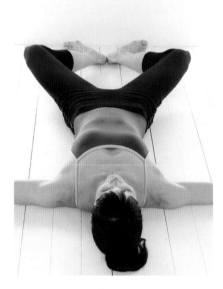

Key:	*Demi-plié* (a half knee bend)

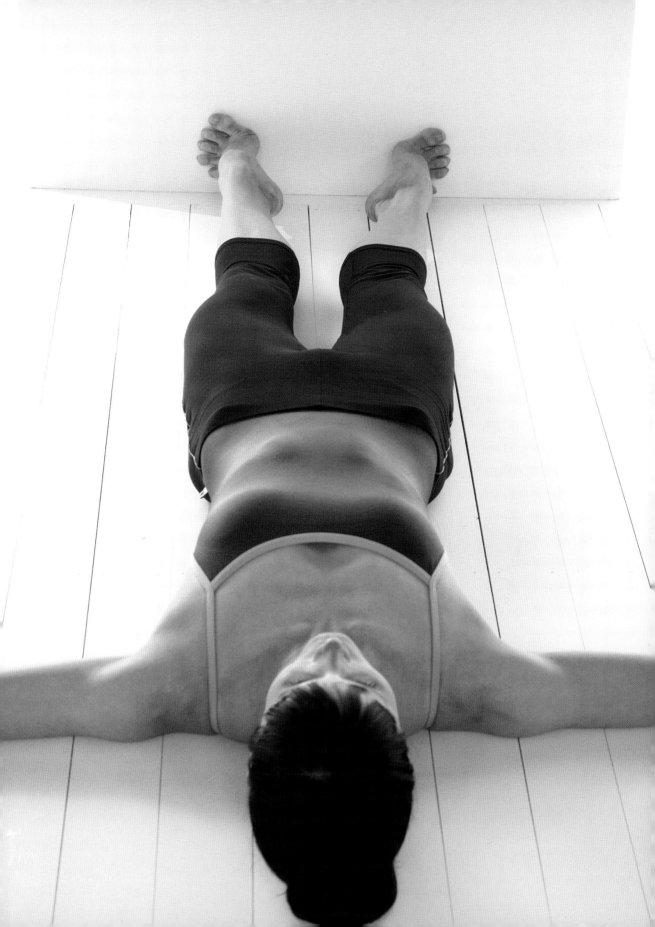

Plié relevé à la seconde (a knee bend followed by a rise to the balls of the feet in second position)

Step one: Get into the starting position for the floor barre.

Step two: Slide your legs out to second position.

Step three: Do a *demi-plié*, keeping your feet in second.

Step four: When your legs straighten, push on to the balls of your feet. Return your feet to second position where your feet are flexed.

Move back to the wall and repeat six times.

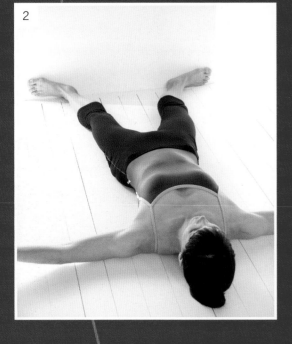

2

Key: | *Demi-plié* (a half knee bend)

Works: | Your feet, thighs and calves

2

3(i)

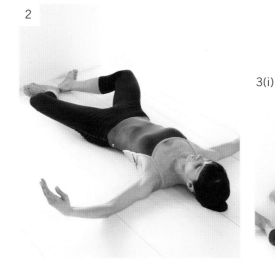

Plié tendu devant (a knee bend with a brushing movement of the foot in front)

Tendu means literally 'to brush'. With *tendus*, the heel always moves first. A good tip I use is to imagine my heel pushing a pile of sand forwards along the wall as I brush upwards or outwards.

Step one: Move back towards the wall and get into the starting position for the floor barre.

Step two: Do a *demi-plié*.

Step three: When your legs return to first position, *tendu devant* (brush in front) your right foot up the wall, keeping your heel on the wall as long as possible. Imagine you are pushing sand with your heel in a straight line up the wall.

Step four: At the top of the movement, your heel will naturally lift off the wall and, as this happens, point your foot so your toes don't lose contact. Using your toes to lead you back, slide your foot back down the wall to first position.

Repeat five times on each leg.

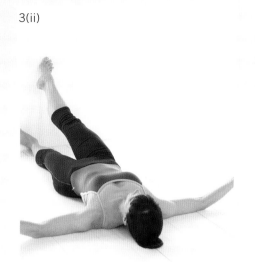

Key: | *Demi-plié* (a half knee bend)

Tip: | The supporting leg, hip
and tailbone must stay
rooted on the floor as
the opposing leg rises along
the wall and into the air

Works: | The muscles in the feet,
the hamstrings and calves

Plié tendu à la seconde (a knee bend with a brushing movement of the foot to the side)

Step one: Stay against the wall and get into the starting position for the floor barre.

Step two: Do a *demi-plié*, and then *tendu à la seconde* your right foot (brush your right foot out to second position) until your heel naturally comes off the wall. Now point your foot. Don't let your toes lose contact with the wall.

Step three: Using your inner thigh and drawing in with your heel, bring your foot back to first position.

The whole movement should last four counts. Repeat five times on each leg.

Tip: Do not lift your supporting hip at all and keep your hips level at all times

Works: Your inner thighs and glutes

2i

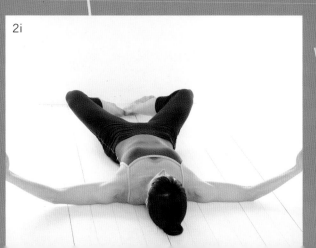

Key: | *Demi-plié* (a half knee bend)

Tendus

Tendus will make your feet and legs very toned and help you to develop a beautiful look to your feet. They're also very good for defining your calf muscles and thighs.

Tip:	There should always be a brushing sensation, but make sure your toes don't come off the wall as you do this
Works:	Your inner thighs, hamstrings and feet

Key:	*Tendu devant* (a brushing movement of the foot in front)

left leg repetition of a **tendu devant**

Tendu (a brushing movement of the foot)

This exercise is in three parts, but should be performed as one movement in six counts.

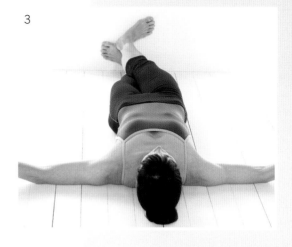

Step one: Get into the starting position for the floor barre.

Step two: *Tendu devant* your right foot by brushing it up the wall, leading with the heel until it lifts off. Point your foot, and then bring it back down to first position. Don't let your foot lose contact with the wall.

Step three: *Tendu devant* your foot up the wall again. Point your foot, but this time draw your heel back to fifth position (the right heel should be against the toe joint of the left foot, and knees should be on top of each other).

Step four: From fifth position, *tendu devant* your right foot back up the wall again, pointing the foot, then draw it back down to first position. Keep your leg straight throughout this entire movement.

Repeat on the left leg.

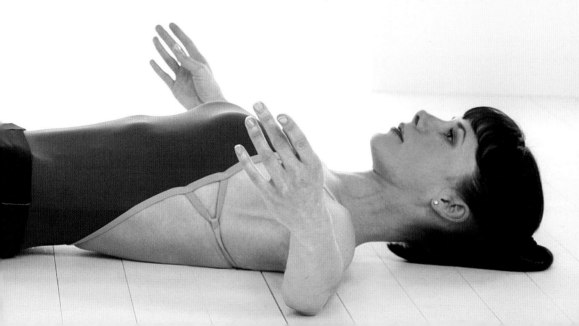

Keep your knees straight when doing *tendus* and don't let the knees bend – this is a mistake many dancers make at the barre. This exercise is also in three parts, but should be performed as one movement in six counts.

Tendu à la seconde (a brushing movement of the foot to the side)

Step one: Get into the starting position for the floor barre.

Step two: *Tendu à la seconde* your right foot by brushing it out and along the wall to second position. Let only your heel lift off at the end, then point your foot.

Step three: Draw your foot back to fifth position using your inner thighs.

Step four: *Tendu à la seconde* your right foot along the wall again back out to second position, point your foot, then draw it back to first position.

Repeat on the left leg.

Tips: Keep your inner thigh engaged at all times to help bring the leg back. Do not let your hips roll as you move and keep your supporting leg still as you *tendu* in second position

Works: Your inner thighs and feet

Key: *Tendu à la seconde* (a brushing movement of the foot to the side)

1

2

3

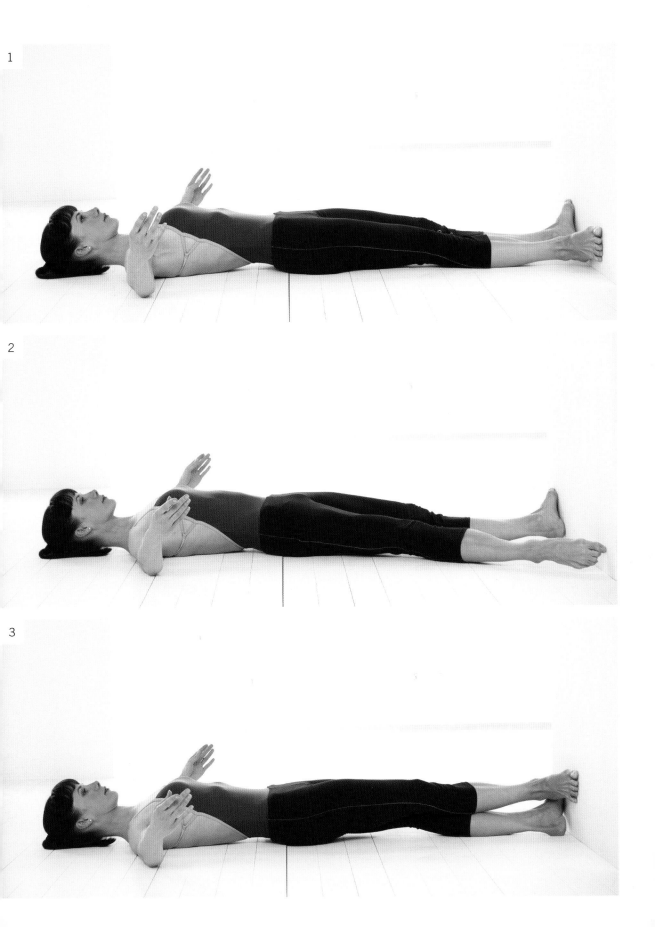

Glissés

Glissés are faster than tendus and make your ankles and toes strong, as well as help you to develop speed in your feet. This is vital for dancing, especially for allegro work (faster dance moves) and the jumping steps.

Glissé
(a sliding movement of the foot in which it comes off the floor)

Step one: Get into the starting position for the floor barre.

Step two: Tendu devant your right foot up the wall, leading with your heel. When your heel naturally lifts off, point your toes and lift them away from the wall by about two inches, then bring your foot back down to first position.

Step three: Repeat the movement again, but this time return your right foot to fifth position.

Step four: Repeat one last time and return to first.

The whole movement should last three counts. Repeat on the left leg.

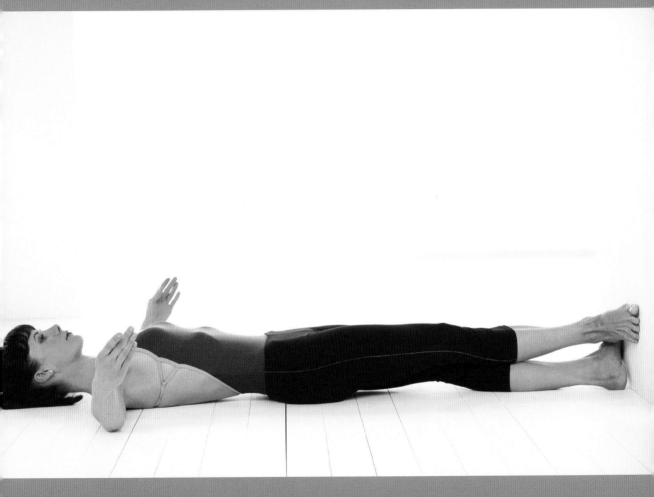

Works: | Your hamstrings and calves

Key: | *Tendu devant* (a brushing movement of the foot in front)

Glissé à la seconde
(a sliding movement
of the foot to the
side in which it
comes off the floor)

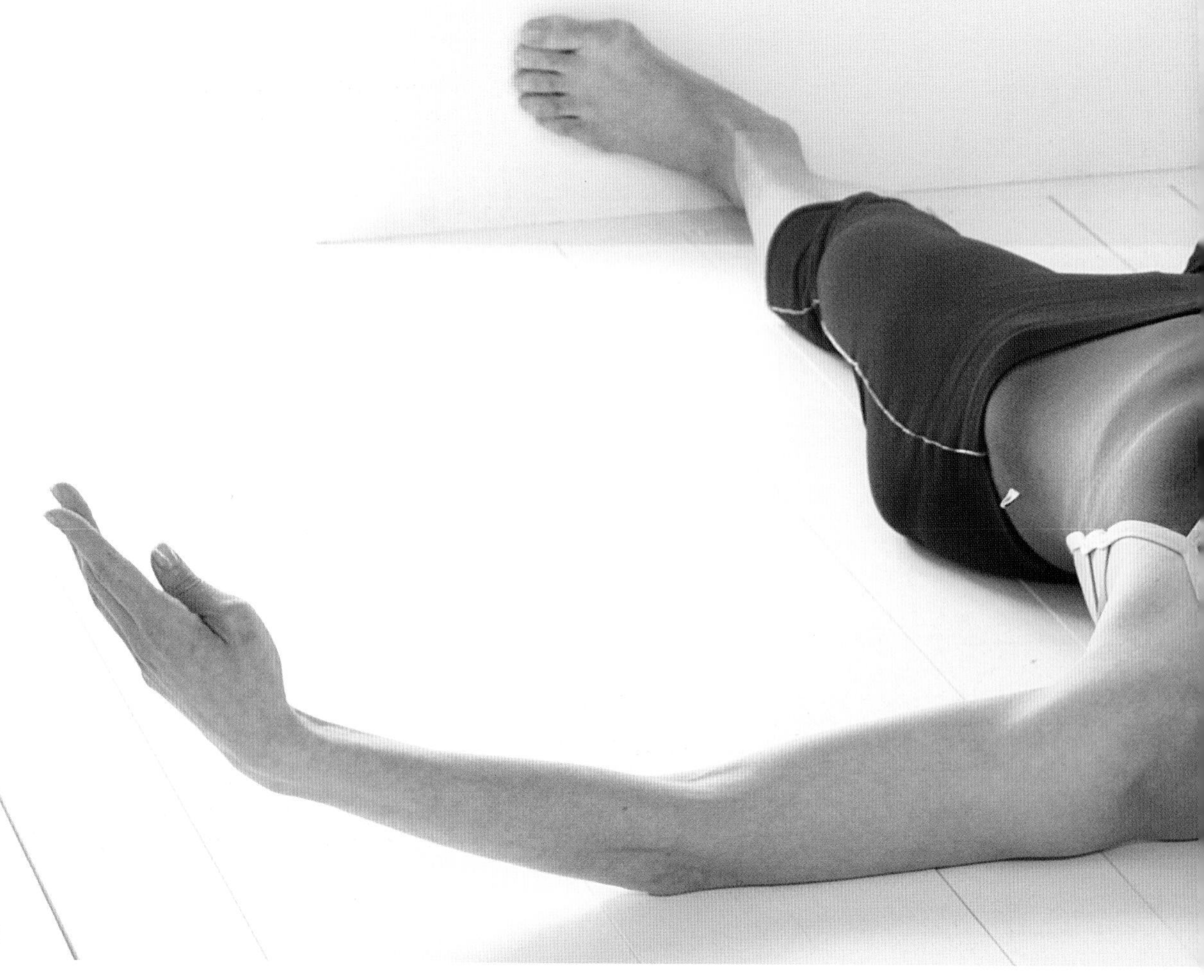

Step one:	Get into the starting position for the floor barre.
Step two:	*Tendu à la seconde* your right leg out to second position, leading with your heel until it naturally lifts off the wall. Point your toes and lift them away from the wall by about two inches. Using your inner thigh, draw your leg back to first position.
Step three:	Repeat the movement, but this time return to fifth position.
Step four:	Repeat again and return to first.
	The whole movement should last three counts. Repeat on the left leg.

3

Tip: When doing moves at a faster pace, always remember to keep your stomach muscles engaged.

Key: *Tendu à la seconde* (a brushing movement of the foot to the side)

Relevé

Ballet dancers go *en pointe* (on point) hundreds of times in a performance. *En pointe* is often an extension of the *relevé* because when you do a *relevé*, you transfer all your body weight up on to the balls of your feet. If you were to continue transferring that weight through the feet to the very ends of your toes, you'd be *en pointe*. However, this is a very advanced technique, so never try it standing if you're not a dancer.

Tip:	Imagine the rise upwards starts at your knees and goes through your calves to your toes
Works:	Your calf muscles and feet

Relevé
(a rise to the balls of the feet)

Step one: Get into the starting position for the floor barre.

Step two: Keeping your legs straight, *relevé* (rise to the balls of your feet) by pushing against the wall with your feet.

Step three: Return to first position by lowering your heels, working through each foot. You won't be able to come back to the wall because your body will have naturally moved away when you rose up.

Return to the wall and repeat five times.

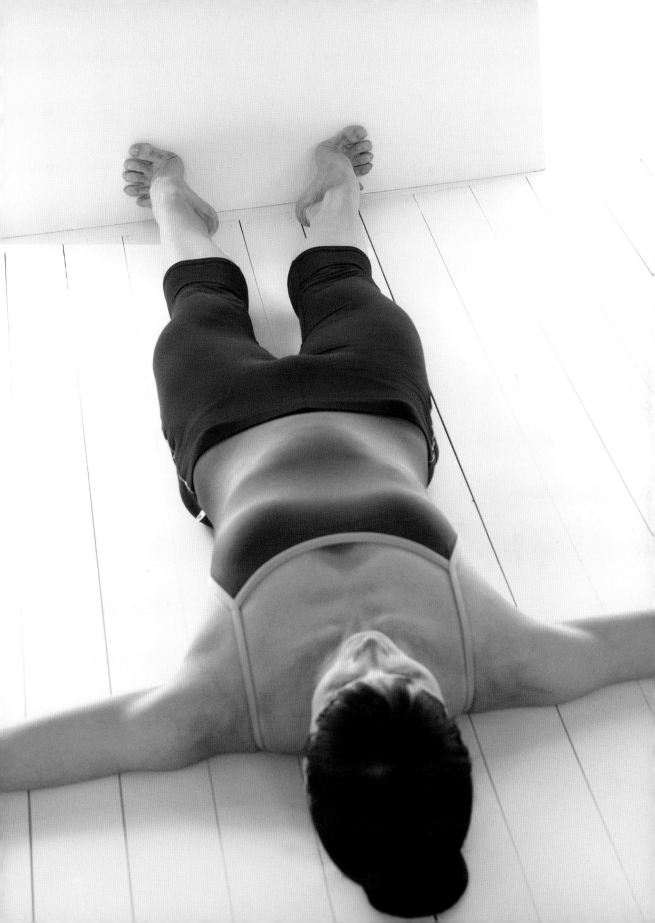

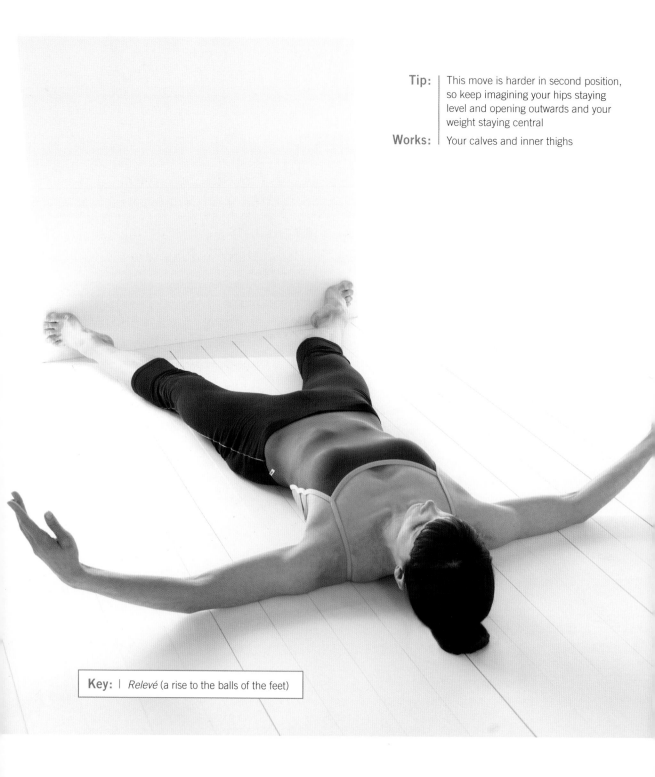

Tip: This move is harder in second position, so keep imagining your hips staying level and opening outwards and your weight staying central

Works: Your calves and inner thighs

Key: *Relevé* (a rise to the balls of the feet)

Relevé à la seconde
(a rise to the balls of the feet in second position)

The *relevé*, which for dancers is done in every position, is crucial to the strength of a ballet dancer's legs because it gives you the strength to support the weight of your body, especially during the jumps. For non-dancers, it's an excellent exercise if you want slim and toned calves.

Step one:	Get into the starting position for the floor barre.
Step two:	Slide your feet out to second position.
Step three:	Keeping your legs straight, *relevé* in second position by pushing against the wall with your feet.
Step four:	Return to second position by lowering your heels, working through each foot.
	Move back to the wall and repeat five times.

Cou-de-pied (a ballet position in which one foot is placed in front of the opposing ankle)

Cou-de-pieds are essential for dancers because this is the action you need to take off for a jump.

Step one: Get into the starting position for the floor barre.

Step two: *Cou-de-pied* by raising your right leg off the floor and, as you do so, bend your knee slightly and turn it outwards. Point your toes and touch your left anklebone before returning to first position.

Repeat four times on each leg.

Works: This move is to create strength in your pointed foot and ankle

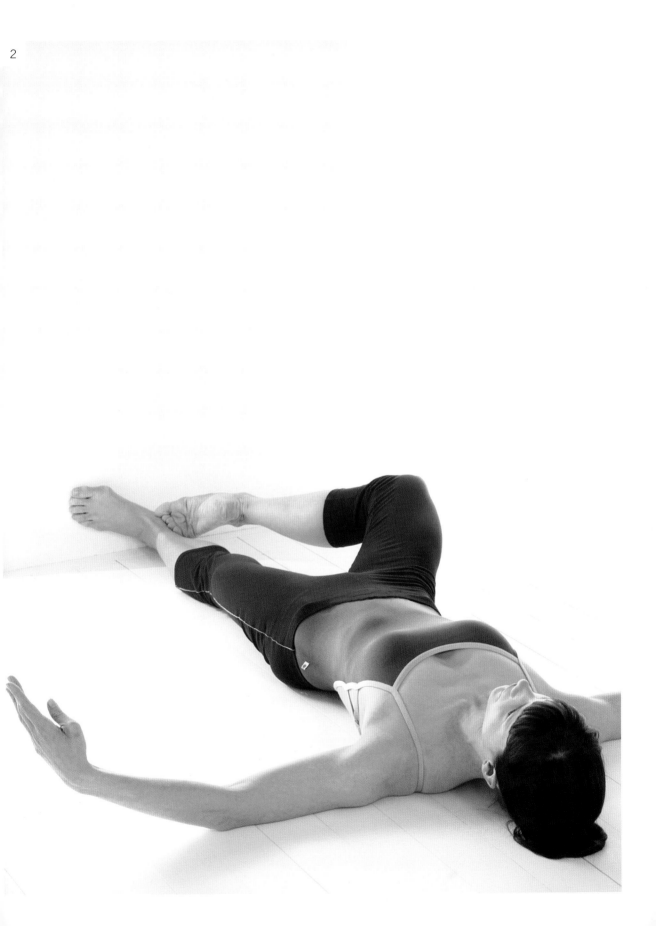

Fondu devant and *fondu à la seconde* (a one-legged knee bend in front and in second position)

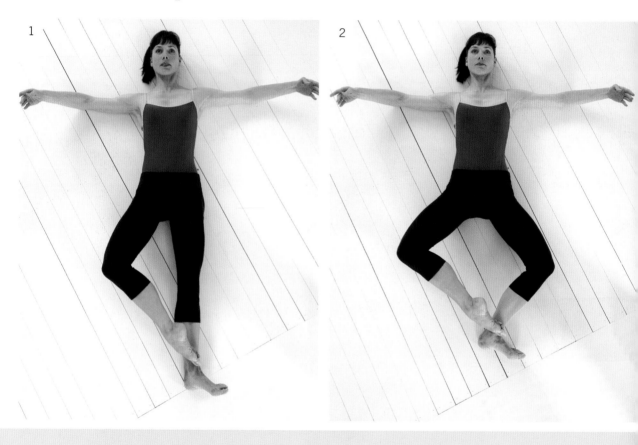

Step one: Move away from the wall and get into the starting position for the floor barre.

Lift your right leg into a *cou-de-pied* (bend your right knee, turn it out and bring your pointed toes to your left anklebone).

Step two: Do a *grand plié*.

Key: *Cou-de-pied* (a ballet position in which one foot is placed in front of the opposing ankle)

Grand plié (a deep knee bend)

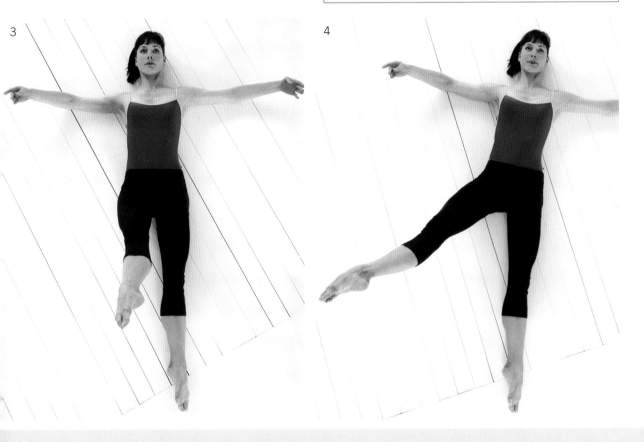

Step three: In two counts straighten both legs and at the same time lift your right leg into the air to a forty-five-degree angle off the floor. Your left foot should also be pointed.

Step four: In another two counts bring your legs back into a *cou-de-pied*. Do another *grand plié*, straighten both legs and, this time, again in two counts, swing your right leg outwards to second position at a forty-five-degree angle. Take two counts to return your legs to first position.

Repeat on the opposing leg.

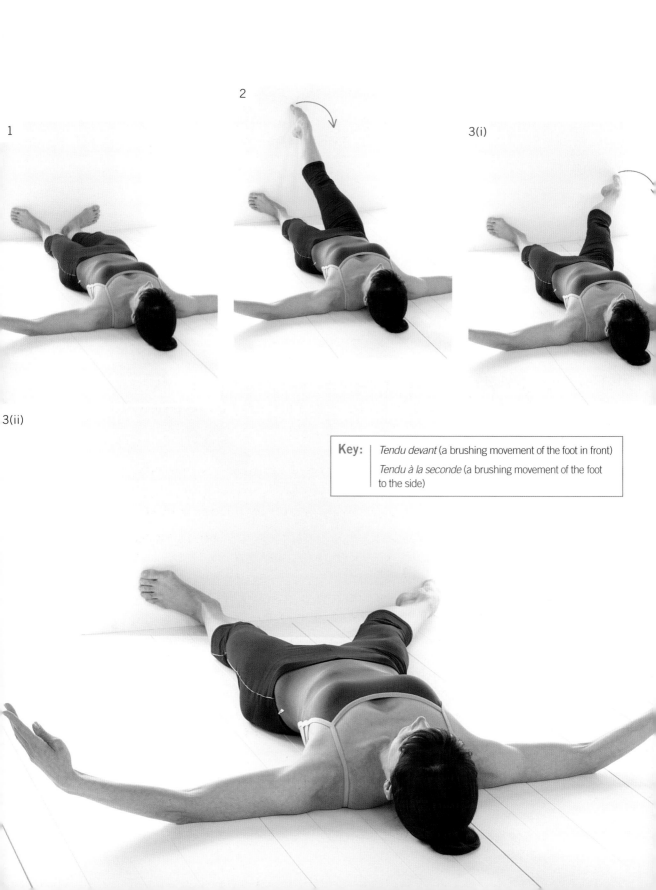

1

2

3(i)

3(ii)

Key: *Tendu devant* (a brushing movement of the foot in front)

Tendu à la seconde (a brushing movement of the foot to the side)

Tip:	This is a strengthening move so it's important to keep the supporting leg rooted
Works:	Your thighs, glutes, hamstrings and calves. This is a full lower body workout

Rond de jambe à terre
(a semicircle drawn by the foot on the floor)

This move also focuses on the rotational movement in the hip socket. When dancers do the standing version of *rond de jambe*, the leg is taken all the way back into a half circle off the floor, but in this version, just take the leg to a point that feels comfortable.

Step one:	Move back to the wall and get into the starting position for the floor barre.
Step two:	*Tendu devant* your right foot by brushing it up the wall in front of you, leading with the heel and pointing the toes when they lift off at the end.
Step three:	Then do a *rond de jambe* (a semicircle drawn by the foot) by sweeping your leg outwards and down the wall to second position. Keep your leg straight and foot pointed.
Step four:	Using your inner thigh, draw your leg back along the wall to first position and repeat the whole movement two more times.
Step five:	Then, in reverse, *tendu à la seconde* your right foot by brushing it out to second position. Keeping your leg turned out, make an opposing arc up along the wall with pointed toes, bringing your leg back down to first position. Repeat the reverse movement another two times.
	The movement for each direction should take three counts: one count to brush your leg upwards, one for the arc and one for back to first position. Repeat on the opposing leg.

Rond de jambe en l'air
(a semicircle drawn
by the foot in the air)

This move is excellent for stability and core strength, something all dancers need, but it can be quite hard at first. To help support yourself, keep pulling navel to spine to make sure the supporting leg doesn't move. In the dancer's version of this, we actually make a circle in the air in second position and our leg comes off the floor, which is why it's called *rond de jambe en l'air*.

starting position for the floor barre

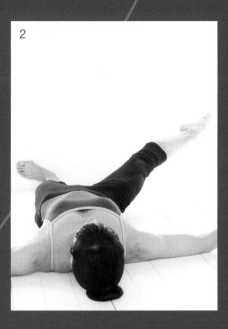

Tip: This is a good ballet beginner's exercise, but you need some knowledge of Pilates to do it. Make sure you do the Pilates short programme before this and don't do it if you find you are wobbling

Works: Your abdominals and all leg muscles

Step one: Get into the starting position for the floor barre.

Step two: Brush your pointed right foot up and out along the wall to second position, letting it lift off the wall about two inches.

Step three: *Ronde de jambe* your leg by making a semicircle in the air: bend your leg and bring your pointed foot to the centre of your left calf, then round your leg back out to second, making an oval.

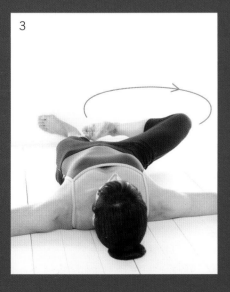

Step four: Draw your leg back to first position using your inner thighs.

The whole movement should take three counts: one to brush your leg upwards and lift off, one to make the arc and one to draw your leg back to first. Repeat once on each leg.

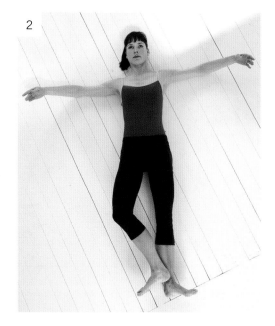

2

Frappé devant
(a forward striking movement with the foot)

The purpose of the *frappé* is to build strength and to sharpen the reflexes in our feet and lower legs so that this move becomes second nature and we can move our feet fast in the right way without thinking.

Step one:	Get into the starting position for the floor barre.
Step two:	Bring your right heel up to rest on the supporting leg's ankle joint. Your right knee should be pointing outwards and your foot turned out and flexed.
Step three:	Keeping your foot flexed and upper leg stable, *frappé devant* by brushing the ball of your foot up the wall in front of you until your leg is straight with pointed toes. Imagine you are striking a match with the ball of your foot.
Step four:	Lower your foot until it is once again resting on the supporting leg's ankle joint, flexed and turned out.
	The whole movement should last four counts: two for raising the leg and two for lowering. Repeat four times.

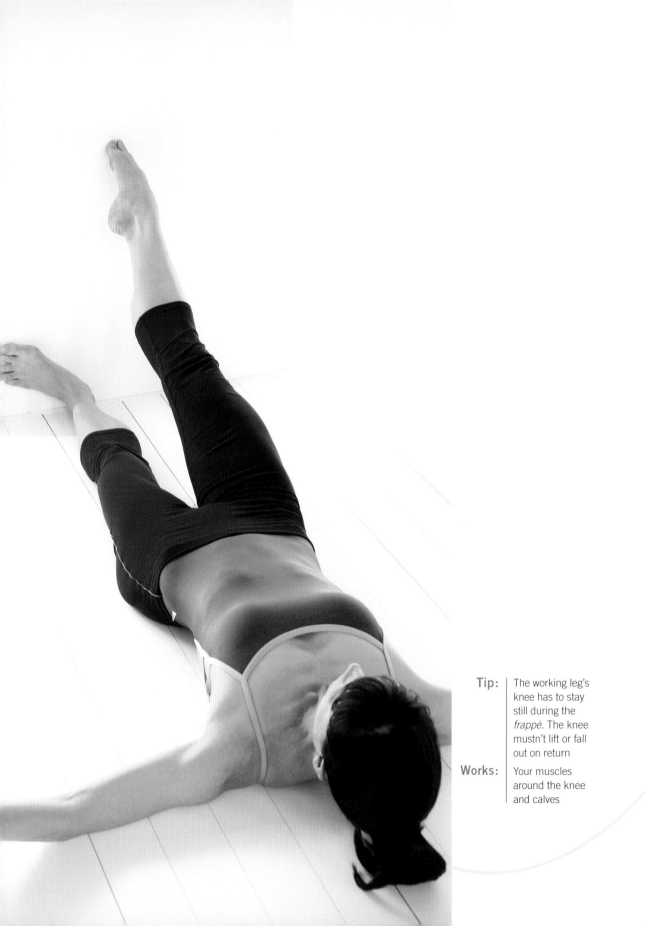

Tip: The working leg's knee has to stay still during the *frappé*. The knee mustn't lift or fall out on return

Works: Your muscles around the knee and calves

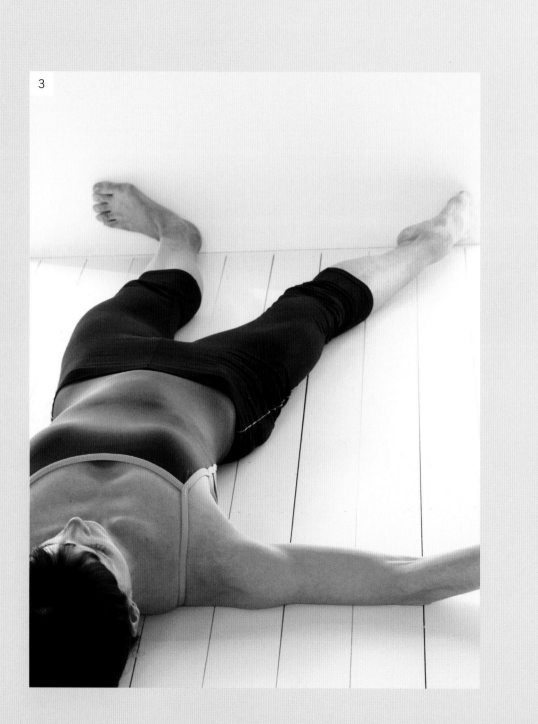

3

Frappé à la seconde
(a striking movement with the foot in second position)

Step one: Get into the starting position for the floor barre.

Step two: Bring your right heel up to rest on the supporting leg's ankle joint. Your knee should be pointing outwards and your foot turned out and flexed.

Step three: Keeping your foot flexed and upper leg stable, *frappé à la seconde* by brushing the ball of your foot in a striking movement out along the wall to second position until your leg is straight with pointed toes.

Step four: Using your inner thigh, bring your foot back to rest on your left ankle joint, flexed and turned out.

The movement should last four counts: two for striking outwards and two for drawing back in. Repeat four times.

Adagio (a slow movement)

Don't feel worried if you can't do an *adagio* straight away, because it's a progression exercise. If a ninety-degree leg lift is too difficult, aim for forty-five degrees to begin with. After a few weeks of doing the floor barre workout, you should be able to achieve the full movement easily.

Step one: Stay against the wall and get into the starting position for the floor barre.

Step two: Point your right foot and draw it up your left leg to rest on the knee. Your right knee should point outwards.

Step three: Leading with the heel and keeping the leg turned out, slowly straighten your right leg in front of you so it's raised at an angle of forty-five to ninety degrees to your supporting leg, with toes pointing to the ceiling. This movement should last two counts.

Step four: Hold in this position for two counts, then, in a slow, controlled movement lasting another two counts, bring the leg back down to first without bending it.

Swap legs.

Tips: Think of making a number four shape when you get into this position. Be careful not to let your tailbone come off the ground when lifting your leg, and don't continue with the exercise if the supporting leg waivers or moves

Works: Your hamstrings and strengthens your core

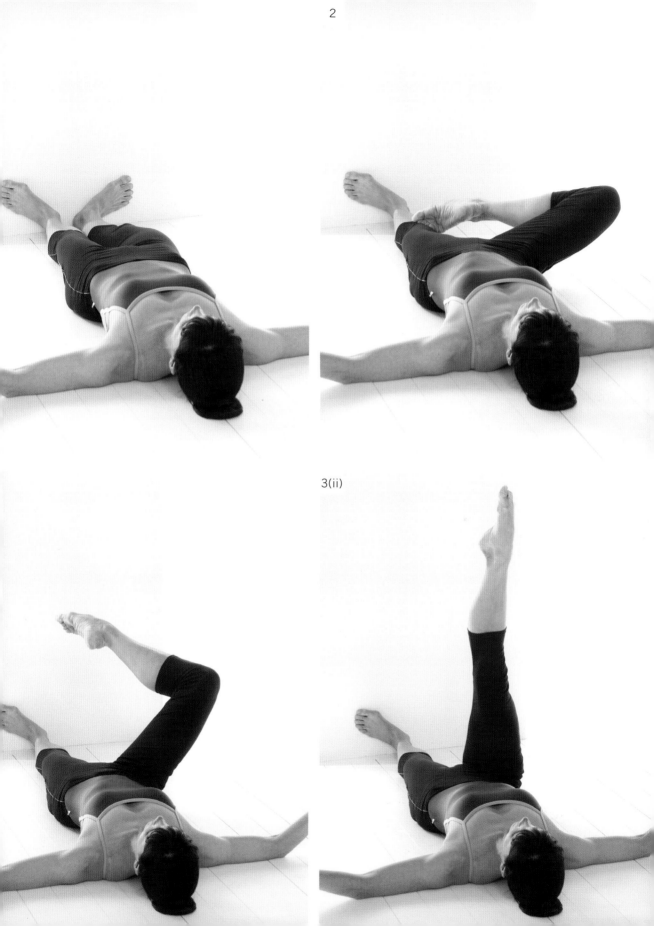

3(ii)

Adagio à la seconde
(a slow movement in second position)

Step one: Get into the starting position for the floor barre.

Step two: Point your right foot and draw it up your left leg to rest on the knee. Your right knee should point outwards.

Step three: Leading with your heel and keeping your leg turned out and toes pointed, slowly straighten your right leg up and outwards to second position so it's at a forty-five to ninety-degree side angle to your supporting leg, with toes pointing outwards. This entire movement should be done very slowly: aim for four counts to lift the leg.

Step four: Hold this position for two counts, then, keeping your leg straight and in a slow, controlled movement lasting two counts, bring your leg down to first position.

Swap legs.

Tip: This is a very hard exercise because the weight of the leg will pull your leg down in the lifted position or will cause your supporting leg to roll inwards. Again, work towards this exercise by focusing on keeping the supporting hip down

Works: Your hamstrings and glutes

Grand battement
(a high throwing kick)

High leg lifts need strength and control and so it's important to work towards these moves over time. The height to which you can take your leg will depend on the flexibility of your hamstrings. Of course, experienced dancers can lift their leg straight up in the air, but this isn't something to aim for. In fact, a forty-five-degree angle is a great start.

Step one:	Get into the starting position for the floor barre.
Step two:	In a kicking action lasting one count, brush your pointed foot up along the wall in front of you and into the air to a forty-five to ninety-degree angle to your supporting leg.
Step three:	Immediately bring the foot back to first position, leading with the heel along the wall.
	Do two kicks on each leg.

Progression:	*Repeat the above movement, but this time kick your pointed right foot up and out to second position so it's at a forty-five to ninety-degree side angle to your supporting leg. Again, do two kicks on each leg.*

Tips:	Keep both legs straight, bellybutton to spine and don't let your back lift off when you raise the leg into the air
Works:	Your hamstrings, thighs and abdominals

Arms

With arm exercises, the upper body should look relaxed at all times. Ballet looks so smooth and effortless because the legs are where all the strength comes from, so we're taught to hold no strain in the upper body.

1

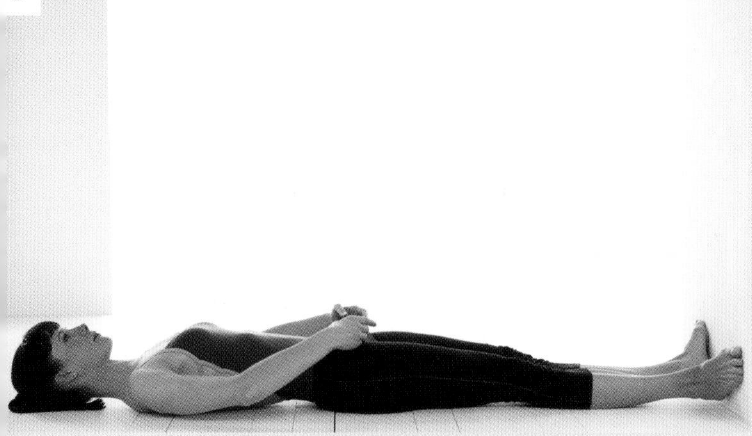

Tip: The shoulders shouldn't lift at all in *port de bras*: the movement comes from the arms moving in the arm sockets

Works: Your lats and opens the chest

2

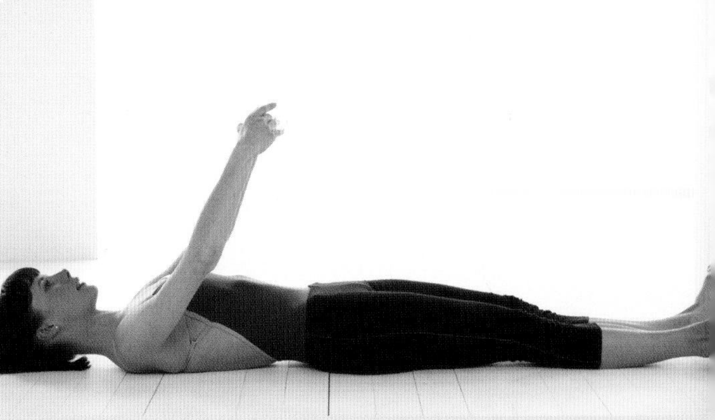

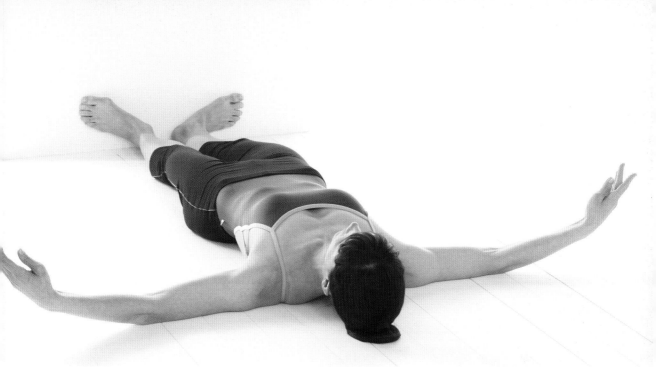

Demi-port de bras
(a half carriage of the arms)

This is a lovely way to open the chest out.

Step one: Lie on your back with your feet in first and your arms in the prepare position (a long oval shape, with your palms resting on your hips just below your pelvis and facing towards you).

Step two: From here, lift your arms in front of your body to first position so that the palms of your hands are facing your navel. Keep your elbows slightly bent (imagine you're holding a large beach ball).

Step three: Leading with your fingers, open your arms out to second position (arms open to the side of your body, just below shoulder height).

Step four: Move your arms back down to prepare position.

Repeat four times in one smooth and continuous movement.

Full port de bras
(a full carriage of the arms)

Step one: Lie on your back with your feet in first and your arms in the prepare position.

Step two: Lift your arms upwards into first position.

Step three: From here, and leading with your fingers, raise your arms to fifth position above your head (but so you can still see your palms without moving your head).

Step four: Open your arms outwards to second position and, keeping the curve in your arms, bring them back to prepare position.

Repeat four times in one smooth and continuous movement.

Works: | Your lats, chest and triceps

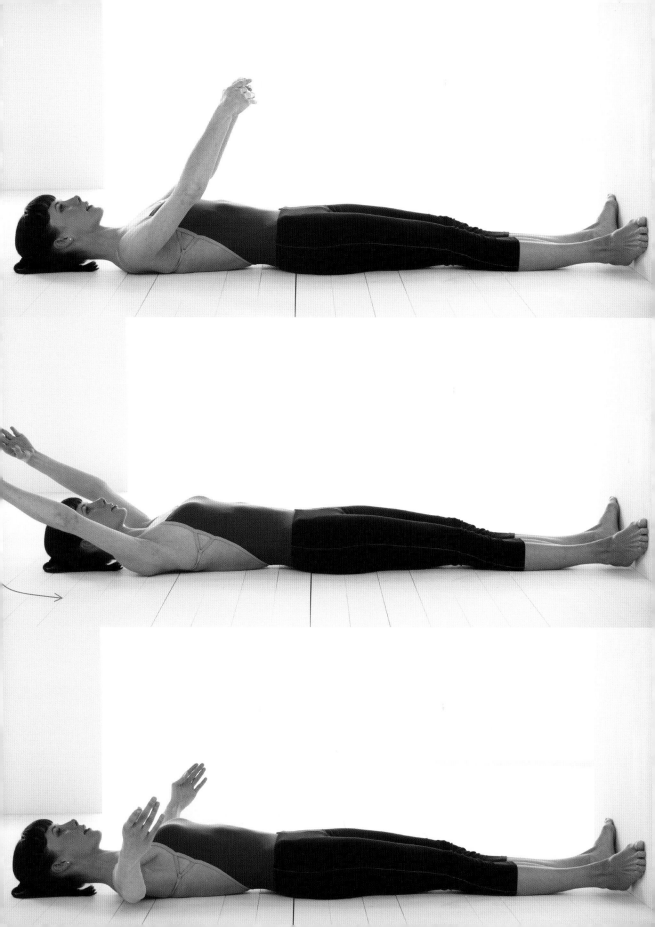

2

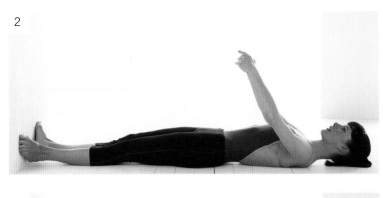

3

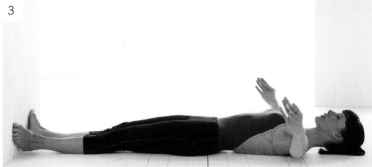

Tip: If your necks hurts or your shoulders lift off, try putting a rolled-up hand towel under your neck for extra support

Works: Your lats, chest and triceps

Reverse full port de bras
(a carriage of the arms in reverse)

Step one: Lie on your back with your feet in first
             and your arms in the prepare position.

Step two: Lift your arms upwards into first position.

Step three: From here, lead out with fingertips to
             second position.

Step four: Then move your arms to fifth position
             and back down to prepare.

             Repeat four times in one smooth and
             continuous movement.

fifth position

THE STANDING BARRE (ADVANCED PROGRAMME)

For anyone who loved doing the floor barre and is eager to get the feel of what it's like to do a standing barre workout, I've put together a less complicated version of the professional dancer's barre. This standing programme represents half the amount of exercises that dancers would normally do in a barre class, but it will give you an idea and feeling of what it's like to exercise like a dancer. When you feel ready to advance to the standing barre, I would do the floor barre workout first as the warm up, then the standing barre as the main programme and then cool down with the stretching programme.

What you need to start

You will need one of the following to hold on
to and use as your 'barre':

- A sturdy stool with a high back
- A kitchen work surface
- A high-backed sofa
- A solid dining room chair with a high back
- Basically, anything sturdy or secured that is waist height

The essential standing barre basics

The five positions of the legs and arms standing up

When moving your legs into ballet positions, you should never feel a pulling in your knees, only in your upper legs and glutes. If you start to feel any kind of strain in your knees, immediately release the position and resume at an angle that feels more comfortable.

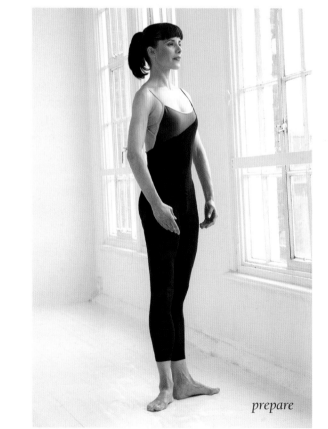

prepare

Prepare

Legs: Stand with your legs turned out, heels touching, your hips facing forwards and your toes pointed outwards.

Arms: Keeping your shoulders pulled down and upper body relaxed, your arms should be slightly curved into a long oval shape with palms near your hips.

First position

Legs: First position for the legs is the same as prepare position: stand tall, pull your navel to your spine and turn out your legs so that your heels are touching. Your hips should be facing forwards and your toes pointing outwards.

Arms: Keeping your shoulders pulled down and upper body relaxed, your arms should be lifted from the prepare position to bellybutton height and held in an oval shape with a gentle bend in the elbows.

Second position

Legs: From first position, slide your pointed right foot out to the side so that heels are a hip-width apart. Lower your heel so that your legs are in line. Your weight should be distributed evenly between both legs and your legs should be turned out and straight.

Arms: From first position, reach through your fingers and open your arms out to the sides of your body just below shoulder height. There should be a slight curve in your arms.

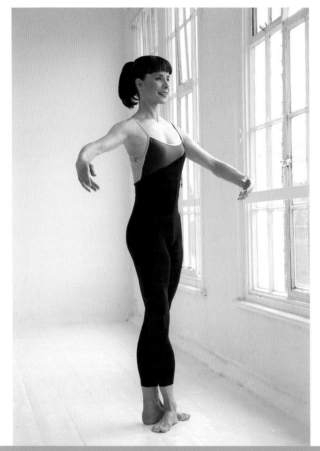

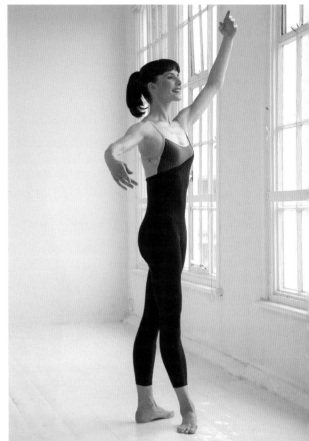

Third position

Legs: From second position, bring your right foot in front of your left foot so that your right heel touches the middle of your left foot just below the toe joint. Knees should be straight, toes pointed outwards and stomach pulled in to help maintain balance.

Arms: From second position, bring your left arm forward so your hand is facing your navel. Keep your arm arced and your fingertips the height of your breastbone. Your right arm should be to the side, with the palm facing forwards.

Fourth position

Legs: From third position, slide your right foot forwards away from your left foot so that it's placed in front of the body (less than a step away). Keep your legs straight and turned out and support yourself from your stomach.

Arms: From third position, lift your left arm over your head, but not so it's directly over it (you need to be able to see your fingers if you raise only your eyes). Be careful not to lift your shoulder, only your arm.

Fifth position

Legs: From fourth position, bring your right foot in front of your left foot, so that your right heel is in front of and touching your left toe. Your knees should be over each other and your hips should not be twisted. Pull up through your knees, thighs and bottom to stand tall.

Arms: From fourth position, lift your right arm to join your left arm above your head, keep your arms rounded and your hands about six inches apart with your palms facing inwards. Again, make sure your shoulders aren't lifted.

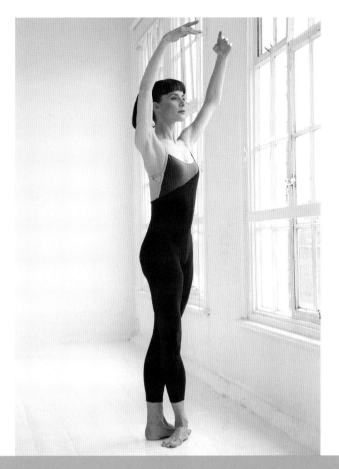

Basic rules

- When standing at the barre (or in the centre), always pull your bellybutton to your spine, keep your legs straight and imagine a string pulling you up from the centre of your head to the ceiling.

- Your arm should be resting on (not gripping) the barre and should be in front of you (not at your side) so you can see your hand if you glance down.

- Always exercise your right side first (holding on to the barre with your left hand). Then, turn around by facing the barre and hold on with your right hand to exercise your left side.

- All exercises start and end in prepare position.

Demi-pliés
(half knee bends)

<table>
<tr><td>Key:</td><td>Demi-plié
(a half knee bend)

Tendu à la seconde
(a brushing movement
of the foot to the side)</td></tr>
</table>

Step one: Stand tall with your left hand resting on the barre at your side and have your feet in first position, turned out from the hip, and your right arm in prepare position. Draw your stomach muscles in. This is your starting position for all standing barre work.

Step two: Keep your pelvis stable and, without lifting your heels off the ground, do a *demi-plié*. As you do this, let your right arm move out to second and come back to prepare as you return upright. As you close your legs together, pull upwards through your inner thighs (do not just straighten the knees). Each movement takes two counts: two for bending your knees and two for straightening up. Do two *demi-pliés*.

Step three: Now *tendu à la seconde* your right foot out to second position with the toe leading the leg (keep your weight on your supporting leg, then transfer on to the working leg so the weight is even). Lower the foot, toe to heel.

1

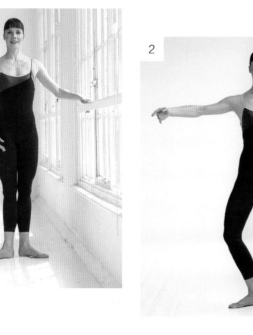

2

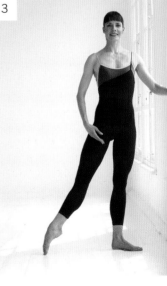

3

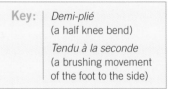

Step four: Do a *demi-plié* in second and, as you do this, let your right arm move out to second and come back to prepare as you return upright. Each movement takes two counts: two for bending your knees and two for straightening up. Do two *demi-pliés* in second.

Step five: Move your feet back into first position by pointing the toes of your right foot and brushing them back along the floor towards your left foot, keeping your leg straight, until your heels meet.

Turn around by turning towards the barre and repeat the sequence on your left side.

Tip: When in first position, only turn out as much as you comfortably can

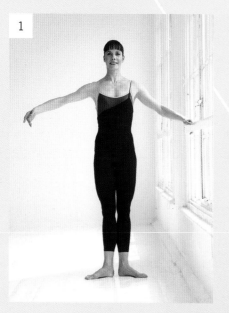

Tendu en croisé
(a brushing movement of the foot in all directions)

Step one: Get into the starting position for the standing barre. *Port de bras* your right arm to second by first moving it to first position, and then out to second.

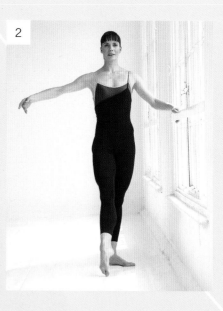

Step two: *Tendu devant* by brushing your right foot out in front of you, guiding with your heel. When your heel starts to come off the ground, point your toes, but don't let them lose contact with the floor. Brush your foot back along the floor to first position until your heels meet.

Step three: Now *tendu à la seconde* by brushing your right foot out to second position, pointing your foot, and then closing it back to first.

4

Tip: Always keep your legs straight and make sure there is no bend in the knees when *tenduing*

Key: *Tendu devant* (a brushing movement of the foot in front)

Tendu à la seconde (a brushing movement of the foot to the side)

Demi-plié (a half knee bend)

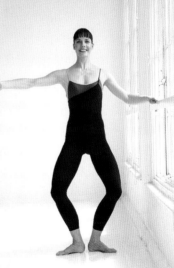

5

Step four: Next *tendu derrière* (a brushing movement of the foot out behind you), point your toes, and then close back to first.

Step five: Finally, do a *demi-plié*, at the same time letting your arm come back down to prepare position as you return upright.

Turn around and repeat on the left side.

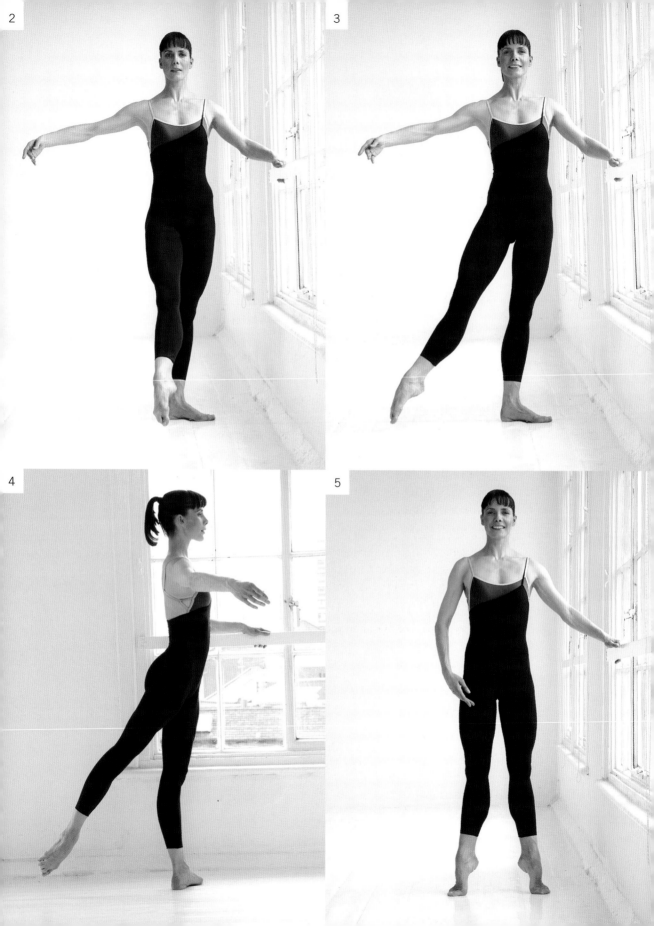

Glissé
(a sliding movement of the foot in which it comes off the floor)

Step one: Get into the starting position for the standing barre. *Port de bras* your right arm to second position.

Step two: From this position, *glissé devant* by sliding your right foot out in front of you until your toe naturally lifts about two inches off the floor in a pointed position. Bring the pointed toe back down to the floor and *tendu* back to first.

Step three: Now *glisse à la seconde* by sliding your foot out to second until your pointed toes lift off the floor (but don't transfer the weight of your body on to your working leg), then *tendu* back to first.

Step four: Next, *glissé derrière* by sliding your foot behind you until your pointed toes lift off the floor. Return your foot to the floor and close back to first.

Step five: Finally, *relevé* (a rise to the balls of the feet) by pulling up through your knees and thighs (your heels will naturally come apart from first position as you do this), and then lower back down to first position, bringing your arm back down to prepare.

Turn around and repeat on your left side.

Key:	*Port de bras* (a movement of the arms from one position to another)
	Tendu (a brushing movement of the foot)

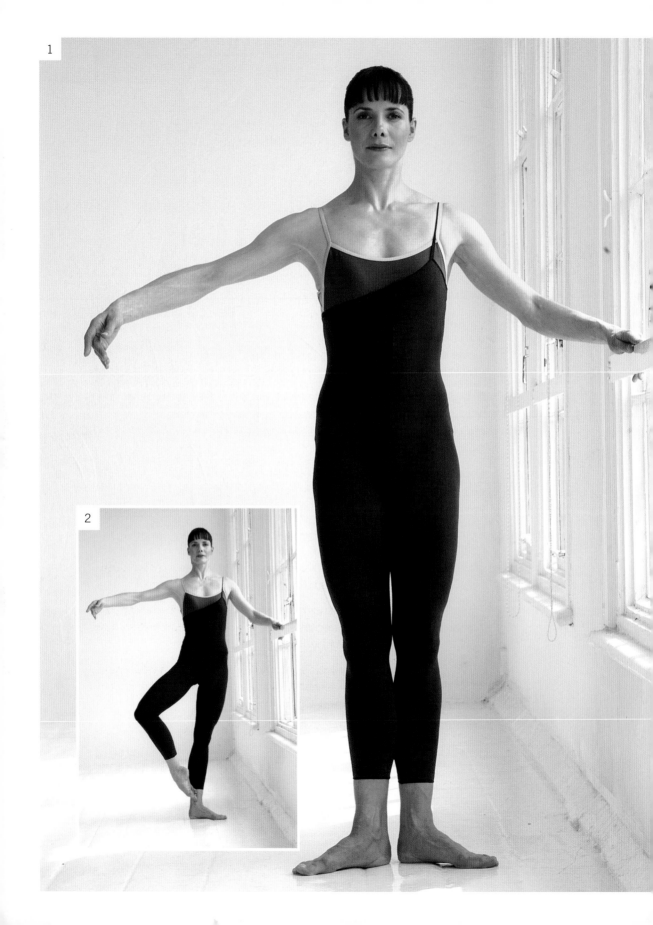

1

2

3(i)

3(ii)

4

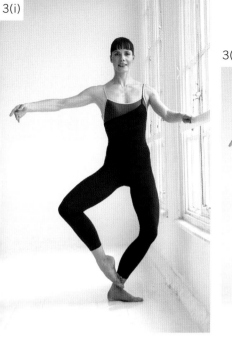

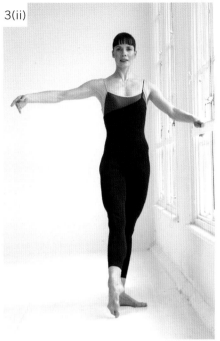

Fondus and rond de jambe
à terre (one-legged knee bends and a semicircle drawn by the foot on the floor)

Step one: Get into the starting position for the standing barre. *Port de bras* your right arm to second position.

Step two: Bring your right foot into a *cou-de-pied* by touching your pointed toes to your left anklebone, ensuring that the heel is forwards.

Step three: In two counts do a *grand plié* and, as you straighten your left leg, *tendu devant* your right leg by extending it out in front of you and pointing your toes.

Step four: Bring your foot back into a *cou-de-pied*.

Tips: Do not let the right hip open out; your hips should stay facing forwards. Pull up through the inner thighs

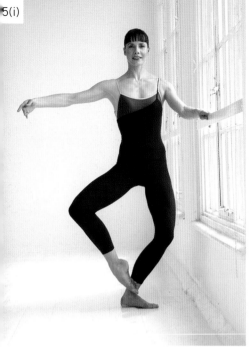

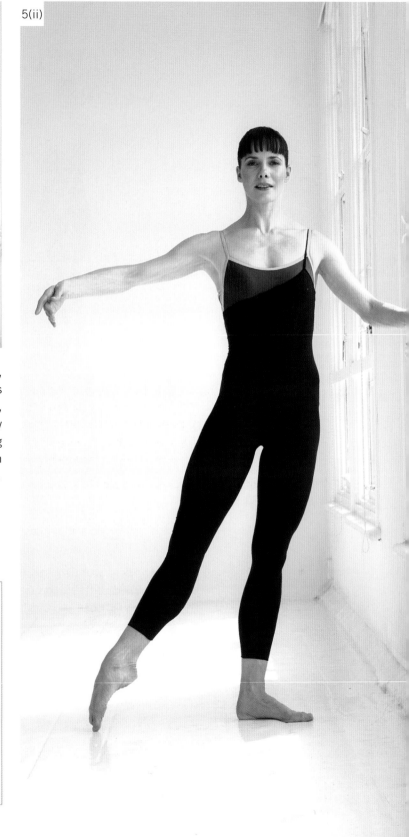

Step five: Again, in two counts, do a *grand plié* and, as your left leg straightens, *tendu à la seconde* by extending your right leg out to second position and pointing your toes.

Key: *Port de bras* (a movement of the arms from one position to another)

Cou-de-pied (a ballet position in which one foot is placed in front of the opposing ankle)

Grand plié (a deep knee bend)

Tendu devant (a brushing movement of the foot in front)

Tendu à la seconde (a brushing movement of the foot to the side)

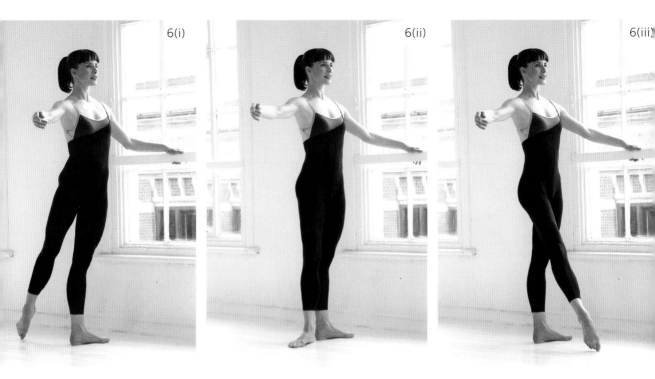

6(i)   6(ii)   6(iii)

Step six: From second position and keeping your pointed toes on the floor and your leg straight, *rond de jambe* (a semicircle drawn by the foot) in one smooth movement. Brush your toes behind you, bring them through to the front (going through first), and then back around to second. Continue it on behind you and finally bring it back to first, lowering your arm back to prepare position at the same time. This whole movement should take four counts.

Turn around and repeat on the other side.

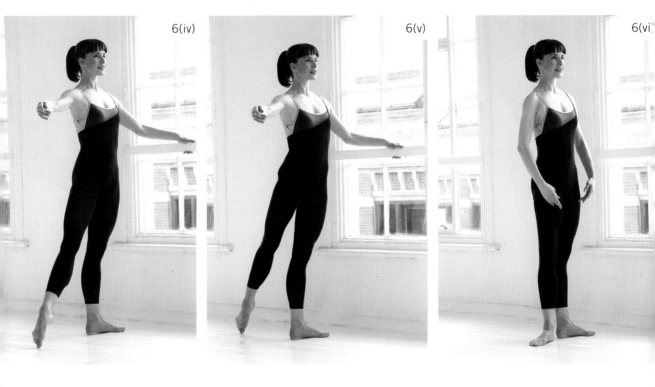

6(iv)   6(v)   6(vi)

2

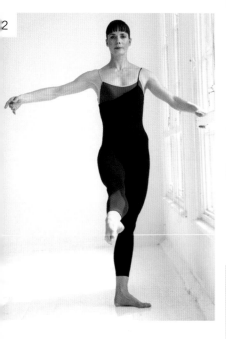

3

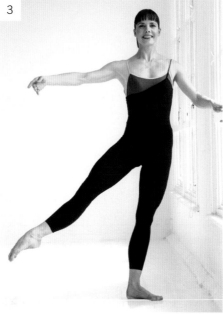

4

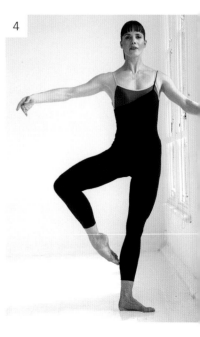

Key: | *Port de bras* (a movement of the arms from one position to another)
Dégagé devant (a brushing movement to the front in which the foot comes off the floor at a forty-five-degree angle)
Dégagé à la seconde (a brushing movement to the side in which the foot comes off the floor at a forty-five-degree angle)

(i)

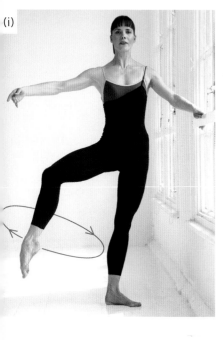

5(ii)

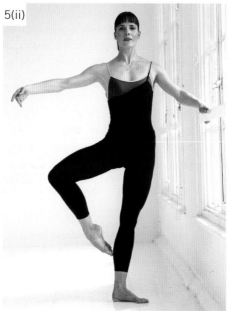

6

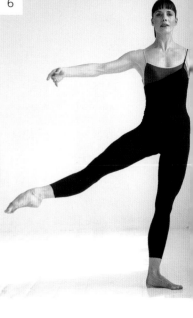

Dégagé and *rond de jambe en l'air* (a brushing movement in which the foot comes off the floor at a forty-five-degree angle and a semicircle drawn by the foot in the air)

Step one: Get into the starting position for the standing barre. *Port de bras* your right arm to second position.

Step two: *Dégagé devant* your right foot out in front of you: lift your leg and move it to a forty-five-degree angle to your supporting leg (about the level of your other knee). Lower your leg back to the floor to first position. Take two counts to raise your leg and two counts to lower it.

Step three: *Dégagé à la seconde* your leg out to second position, lifting it to the side at a forty-five-degree angle (keep your heel and leg slightly to the front of your body when lifting and your weight on your supporting leg). Take two counts to raise it and two counts to lower it, then raise it again.

Step four: From this raised position, and keeping your upper leg stable, bring your pointed right foot to the calf of your left leg.

Step five: From here, *rond de jambe* your right leg in an arc shape in the air by moving your foot forwards, out to the side, then back to the calf.

Step six: Return your leg to the forty-five-degree lift at your side.

Step seven: Repeat the *rond de jambe en l'air* two more times (steps 4–6), and then lower your leg to second position. Brush your foot back into first, at the same time bringing your arm down to prepare position.

Turn around and repeat on the left side.

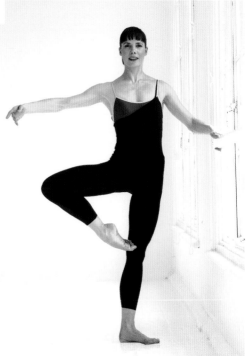

Step one: Get into the starting position for the standing barre. *Port de bras* your right arm to second position.

Step two: Lift your right leg into a *retiré* (one-legged balance) by bending your right knee and keeping your leg turned out, then drawing your pointed toes up your left leg to touch your left knee (think of making a number four with your legs). From here, brush your right foot back down your left leg to first position.

Tips: Do not lift your right hip as you bring your right leg into a *retiré* and make sure your foot is always in front of the knee and not to the side

Retiré and grand battements
(a one-legged balance and high throwing kicks)

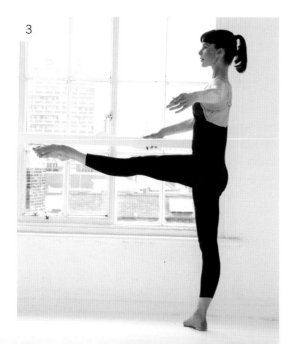

Step three: Next, *tendu devant* your right foot in front of you, keeping your heel forwards, and do a *battement devant* (a kicking movement to ninety degrees in front), being sure to keep your hips stable and back straight. Bring your leg back down to first position.

Step four: Do one more *retiré*, and then a *battement devant*. Bring your leg back down to first.

Tips: Don't let the right hip come up with the leg; it has to stay still. Also, be sure not to let the supporting leg bend to get a higher kick

Step five: Repeat the above process, but this time do a *retiré* and a *battement à la seconde* (a high throwing kick to the side).

Turn around and repeat on your left side.

Tip: | When doing a *battement* in second, have your leg just in front of your body and keep your weight central as you lift your leg

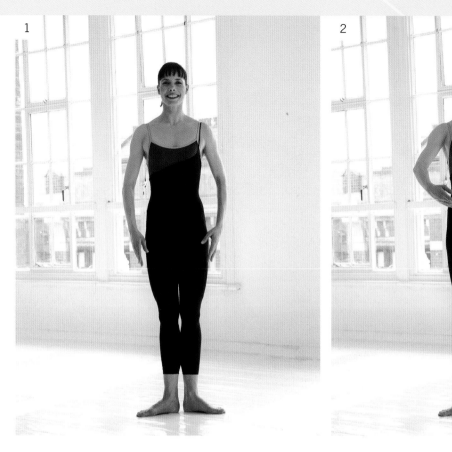

Demi-port de bras (a half carriage of the arms)

Step one: Move away from the barre to the centre of the room. Stand straight with your feet in first and your arms in prepare position.

Step two: From here, lift both arms to first position so that your palms are at bellybutton height and facing towards you.

Step three: Leading out with your fingers, open your arms out to second position (to your side), then lower your arms back down to prepare position.

Repeat twice in a continuous and flowing movement.

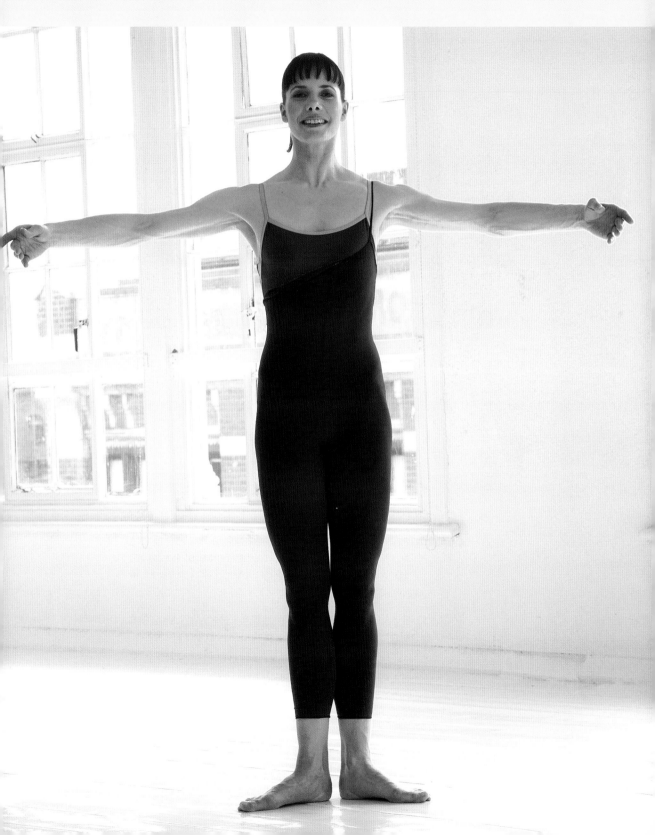

Tips: The arms should never be straight; there should always be a gentle bend in the elbow. The arms should also always be held slightly in front of your body, whether above you or at your sides

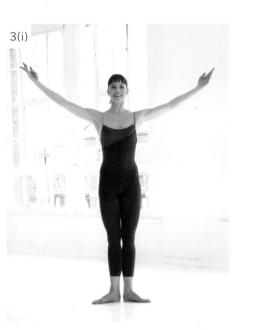

3(i)

Full port de bras
(a carriage of the arms)

Step one: Stay in the centre of the room with your legs in first position and your arms in prepare.

Step two: Leading with your fingers, raise both arms to fifth position above your head (you should still be able to see your fingers if you glance upwards).

Step three: Now, make a semicircle outwards to second position (your palms should face down and there should be a gentle curve in your arms).

Step four: Come back down to prepare position.

Repeat twice in a continuous and flowing movement.

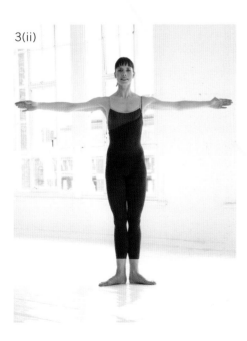

3(ii)

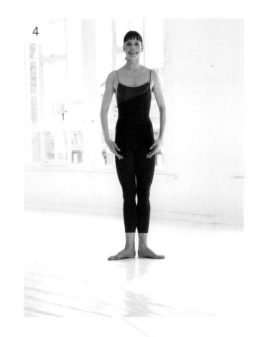

4

2(i)

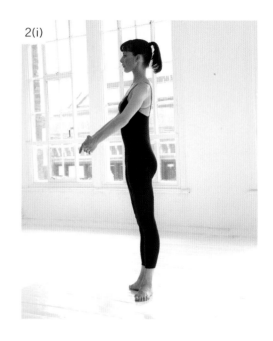

This is a lovely way of warming up the shoulders and giving you flexibility in your upper back.

Arabesque arms

Step one: Stay in the centre of the room with your legs in first position and your arms in prepare.

Step two: Bring your arms up to first position. Then raise your right arm above your head.

Step three: Circle your right arm behind you, turning your palm down as the arm reaches back.

Step four: Bring your right arm back through to first position, at the same time lifting your left arm above your head.

Step five: Circle your left arm behind you, turning your palm down as it reaches back. As you circle it back to first position, move your right arm above your head. Continue this sequence in a continuous and flowing movement.

              Repeat six times.

Tip: Imagine making a windmill with each arm

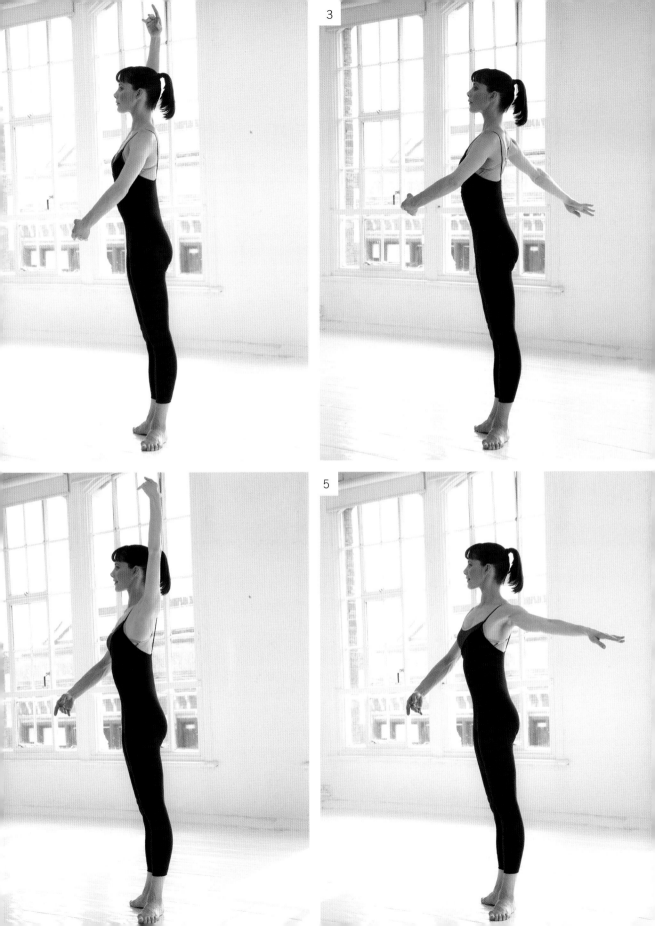

3

Reverse arabesque arms

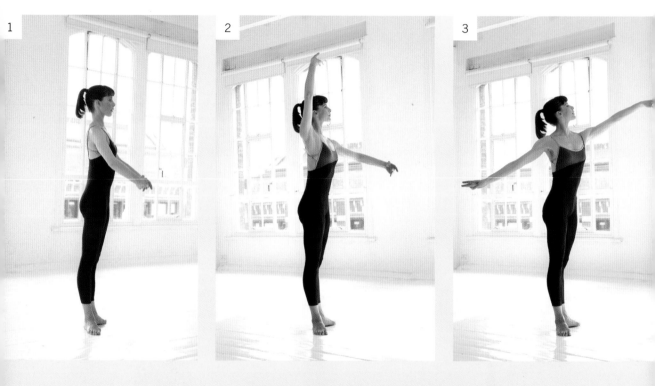

Step one: Stay in the centre of the room with your legs in first position and your arms in prepare.

Step two: Raise your arms to first position, then lift your right arm to fifth position.

Step three: Circle it behind you, and as you do this raise your left arm so that your fingers are at eye level. Both your palms should be facing down.

Step four: Lift your left arm up to fifth position, at the same time bringing your right arm to prepare position.

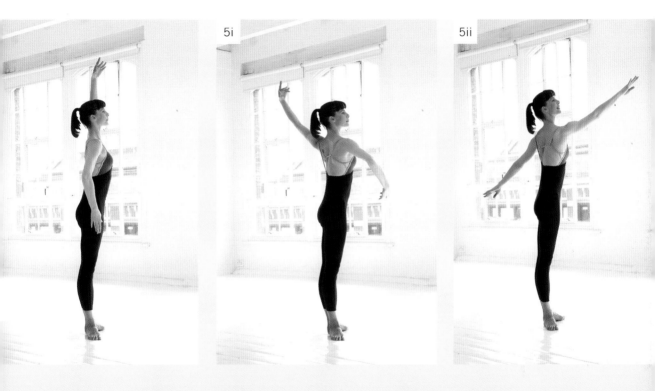

5i 5ii

Step five: Circle your left arm behind you and bring your right arm up to eye level. The left arm should now be straight behind you and the right arm right in front.

Repeat six times in a continuous, flowing movement, imagining you are making a windmill effect with your arms.

Now, reverse the whole action where the arms move forwards rather than backwards (this is very like the front crawl swimming movement). Repeat six times.

Works: | This move gives you breadth and stretch in your upper body and is great for your shoulders and back.

STRETCH

There are three basic types of stretch techniques: ballistic, which is a bouncing movement that has now fallen out of fashion due to safety concerns; a form of active stretching, which is often used in astanga yoga and in certain sports such as athletics; and static stretching, which involves passively stretching a muscle and holding it for around thirty to forty seconds. The latter is the type of stretching in this cool down.

With stretching, it's important to begin with slow, gentle movements because these will make it easier to move into the stretch (rather than throwing your body into a painful position). Never, ever force a stretch or overstretch; your aim is to feel a slight resistance or tension in the muscle, not acute pain. Then, to progress the move, breathe into the stretch. This sounds a silly thing to advise you to do, but many people forget to breathe when they are concentrating during an exercise or when something feels uncomfortable, which means oxygen doesn't get to the muscle and therefore you can't hold the stretch. To breathe correctly, breathe slowly and deeply, in through your nose and out through your mouth. Remember to stretch all your muscle groups and not just the areas that are painful.

Finally, don't compete with someone over how far you can stretch. Our bodies are all made differently and some people are naturally more flexible than others. For instance, as a young dancer I was very supple, but lacked strength to control my movements and so had to teach my body control. No matter how stiff you are, you can teach your body to become more flexible through regular stretching. The goal is not to bend your body into a pretzel or lift your leg behind your ear, but to help your body to relax and let go, which in turn will increase your mobility, build your strength and improve your suppleness. This will decrease your chances of getting injuries and having pains and strains.

Sliding side bends

Step one: Sit on the floor with your legs straight and at approximately a ninety-degree angle (or wider if you're more flexible – but don't force it). Pull your navel to your spine and imagine a string pulling you upwards from the centre of your head.

Step two: Lift your right arm into fifth position, and then bend your body over to the left, allowing your left arm to slide along your left leg to support you. Do not let your supporting hip lift off the floor.

Each stretch should last two counts. Repeat three times on each side.

Stretches: | The side of your body, from hip to neck

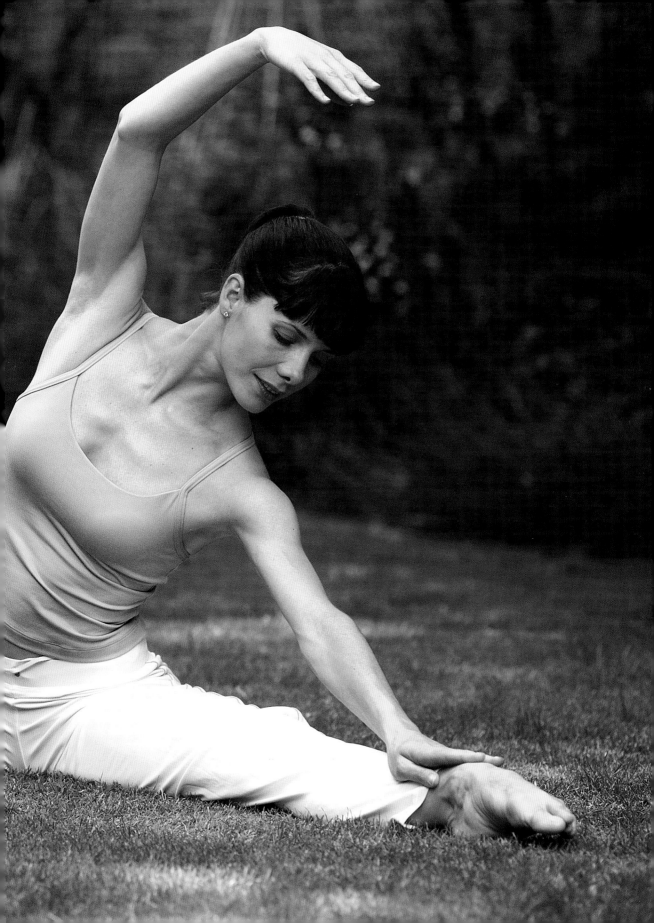

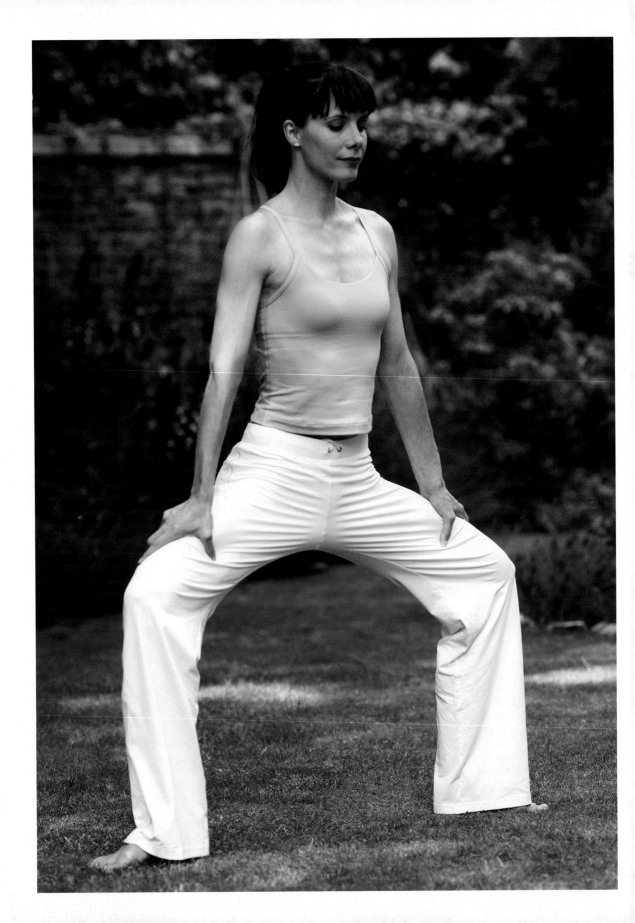

Grand plié in second position

Step one: Stand up and place your legs in a wide position, your feet turned out and your hands resting on the front of your thighs.

Step two: Bend your knees over your feet as far as you can go, keeping the turnout and pulling in your stomach muscles to support you. With your hands on your thighs to support your upper body, make sure your back is straight and hold for two counts.

Step three: Return to the starting position, using your inner thighs to pull yourself up.

Repeat four times.

Stretches: | Your legs, buttocks and thighs

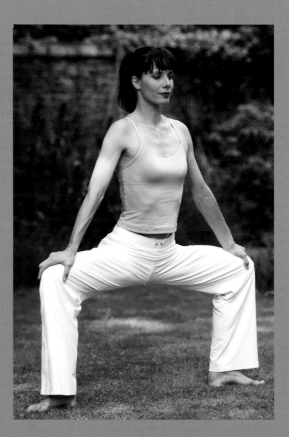

With a dancer's workout the calf muscles will often get quite tight so stretching is very important.

Calf stretch

Step one: Stand with feet together and then step back with your left foot. Bend the right knee slightly, keeping your back straight.

Step two: With hands on hips, push through the heel of your extended leg and tilt your body forwards slightly (imagine there is a straight line running from your heel through to the crown of your head). Hold for thirty seconds and change legs.

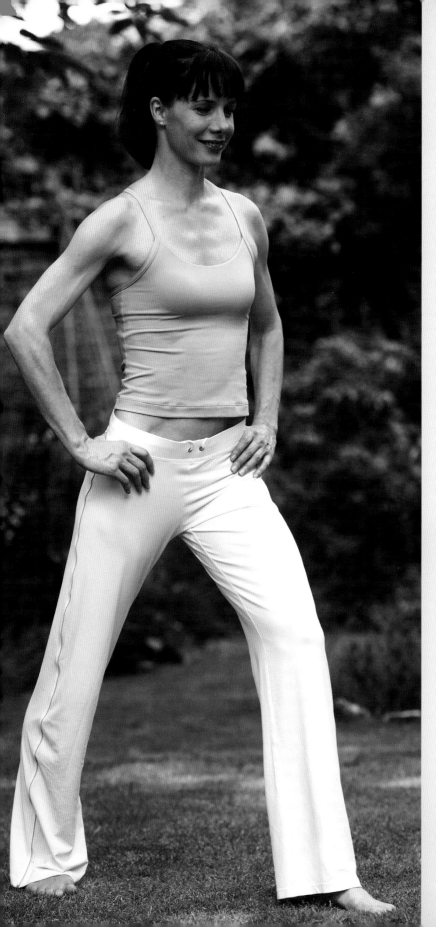

Tip: If you find it hard to balance, do the stretch facing the wall and place your hands an arm's length away on the wall for support

Stretches: Your calves

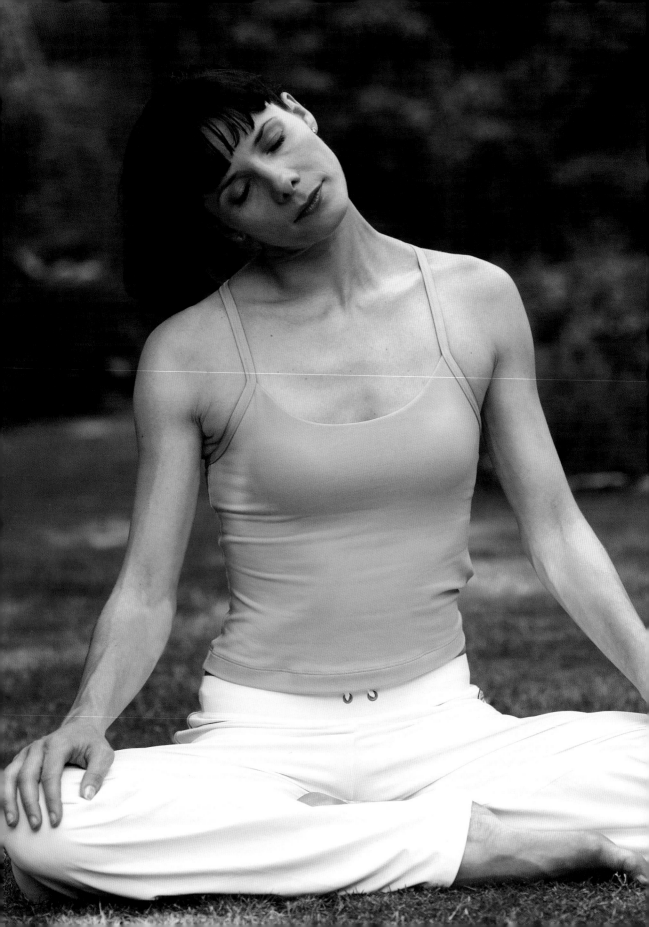

Neck stretch

Step one: Sitting cross-legged on the floor with your stomach pulled in, inhale and drop your head over to the left. Exhale and hold for ten seconds (you should feel the stretch down the right side of your neck).

Step two: Return to the starting position and repeat on the other side.

Step three: Again, return to the starting position and drop your chin to your chest. Exhale and hold for ten seconds.

Repeat the above sequence four times.

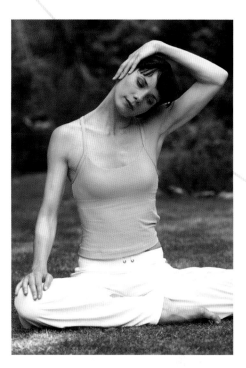

Progression: *As a progression, when you drop your head over to the left, place your left hand over your right ear and let the weight of your hand pull your head towards your shoulder. Repeat on the other side.*

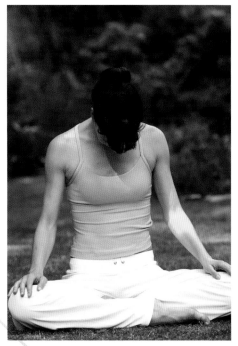

Tip: You should feel a pull along your upper back

Stretches: Your neck, shoulders and upper back

Glute stretch

For dancers, the glutes will always get really tight because of all the turning out we constantly do, so these stretches are a must for us.

Step one: Lie on the floor with your arms at your sides, knees bent and feet hip-width apart.

Step two: Place one foot on the opposing knee. Lift your leg off the floor so it's at a ninety-degree angle.

Step three: Reach forwards and place your hands behind your thigh and pull your leg towards your chest for a thirty-second hold.

Swap legs and repeat.

Tip: Make sure your head stays on the floor
Stretches: Your buttocks and lower back

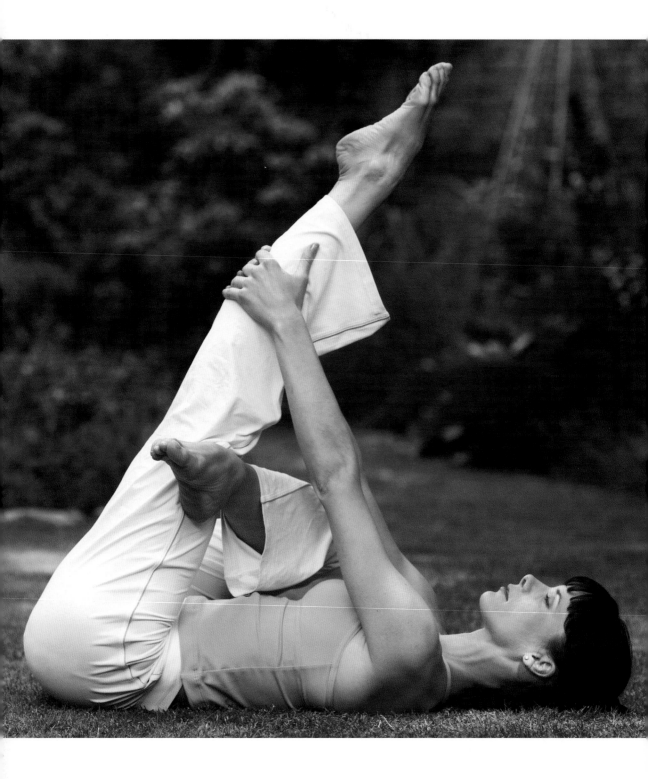

Tip: | Don't worry if you can't pull your leg that close to you. This is a progressive stretch and in time you'll have greater range of movement in your legs

Stretches: | Your buttocks and lower back

Hamstring stretch

Step one: | Lie on your back on the floor with your arms at your sides, knees bent and feet hip-width apart.

Step two: | Place your right foot on your left knee (keep the right knee turned out). Lift your left leg off the floor so it's at a ninety-degree angle. In this position, straighten the left leg.

Step three: | Reach forwards and place your hands behind your left calf (or knee if you can't reach) and pull your leg towards your chest for a thirty-second hold.

Swap legs and repeat.

Tricep stretch

Step one: Sitting cross-legged on the floor, take your right arm above your head. Bend the elbow so the hand falls behind your head, between your shoulder blades.

Step two: Place your opposing hand on your right elbow and gently push the arm down for thirty seconds.

Swap arms and repeat.

Tip: | Keep your shoulder blades pulled down to feel the right stretch

Stretches: | Your tricep muscles below your arms

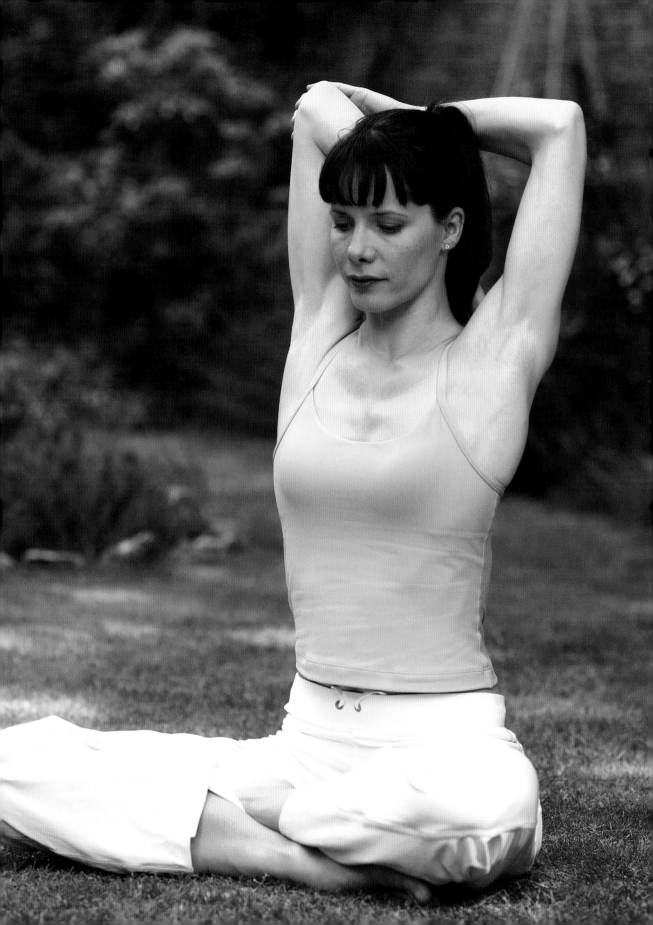

Stretches: | Your triceps and biceps

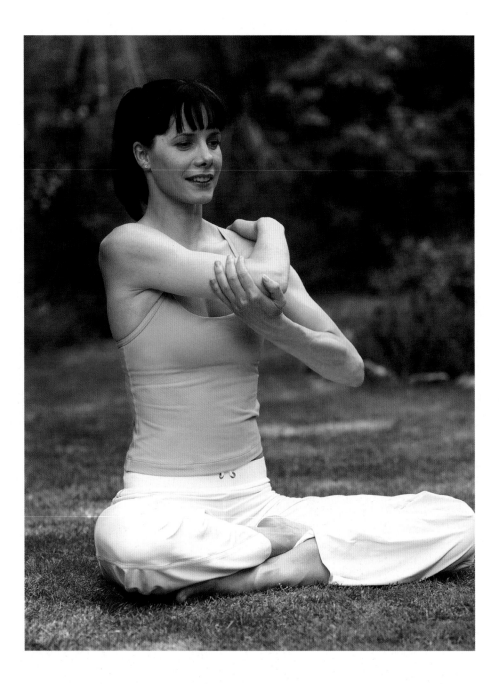

Tip: | Make sure your shoulders are relaxed
as you bring your arm across

Arm stretch

This is a great exercise for people who work in offices.

Step one: Sitting cross-legged on the floor, bring your right arm across your body and place your hand on your left shoulder.

Step two: With the opposing hand, push the right elbow inwards so that the right hand travels over the left shoulder. Hold for thirty seconds.

Swap arms and repeat.

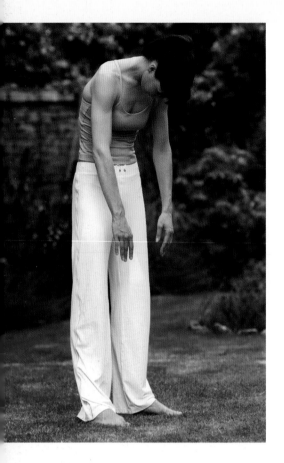

Roll down

Step one: Stand tall with your feet parallel and hip-width apart. Pull your bellybutton to your spine and keep your arms by your sides.

Step two: Inhale and drop your head to your chest. Exhale and, allowing your arms to fall forwards, slowly roll your body down vertebra by vertebra. Keep your legs straight and knees soft, ensuring that you don't rock backwards and forwards. At the bottom of the movement, let your head hang and your hands come as close to the floor as possible.

Step three: Hold for two counts, inhale and, using your stomach muscles, uncurl to the starting position.

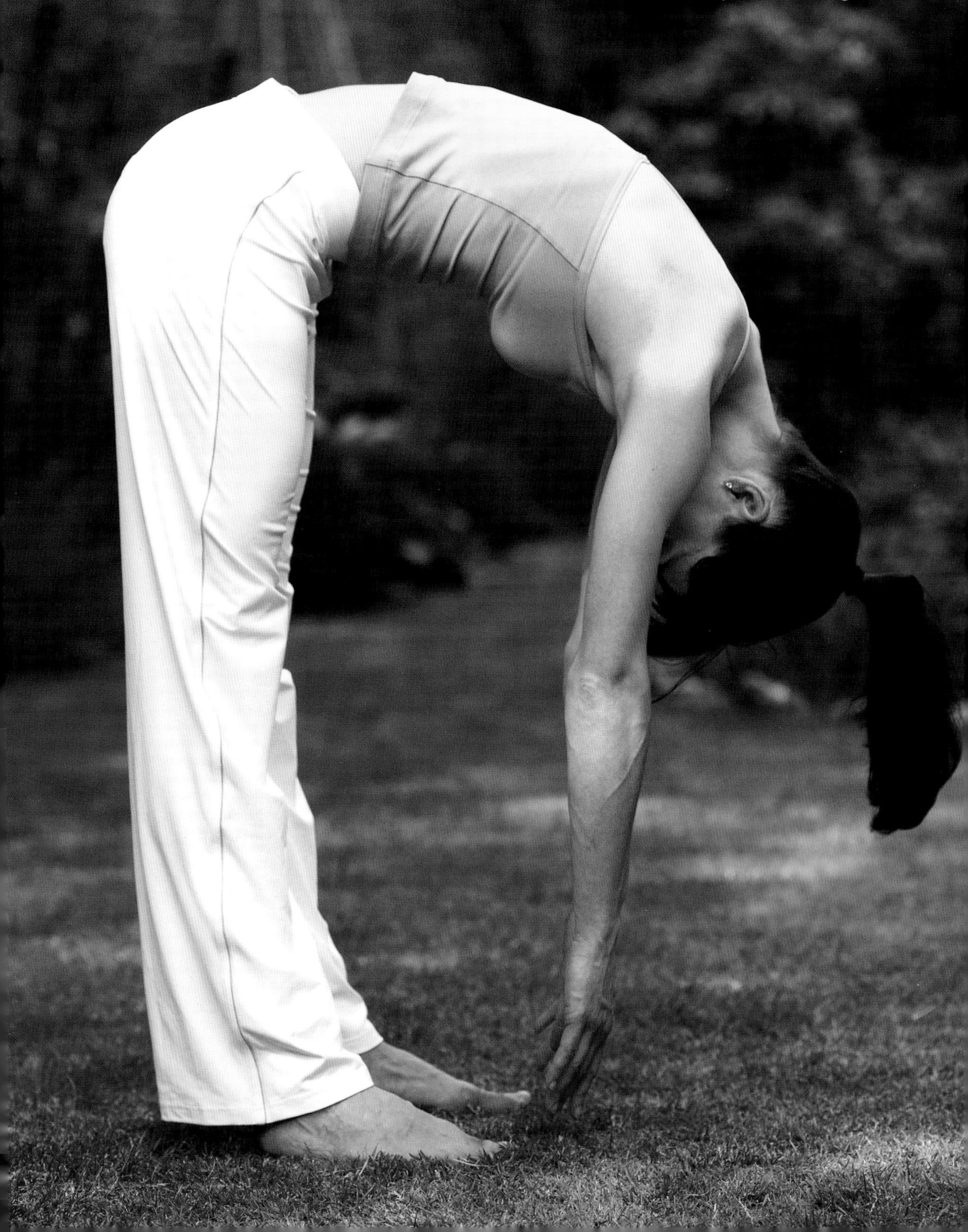

STAYING HEALTHY

In ballet and in life, I find that it's essential to protect your body from injury in any way that you can. For me this means good warm ups, lots of exercise, stretching, Pilates and enough rest (though as any mother knows, this last point can be hard when you have children).

It's not about weight, it's about fitness, and one component of being fit is to have relatively low body fat because fat is not very efficient at burning calories, whereas muscle is. If weight loss is your aim, it's worth knowing that the Pilates, floor barre and stretch workout alone is not going to make you lose weight. While body conditioning helps you lose inches, it's cardiovascular exercise, such as running, walking, cycling and swimming, that helps you to lose fat/weight. If you think ballet dancers are all lucky to be so thin, take a look at how rigorous a ballet is and you'll see why dancers are so lean. For this reason, a healthy lifestyle is an essential factor alongside this exercise programme. To reap the best benefits, I've given some advice below to maximize the effects of the workout.

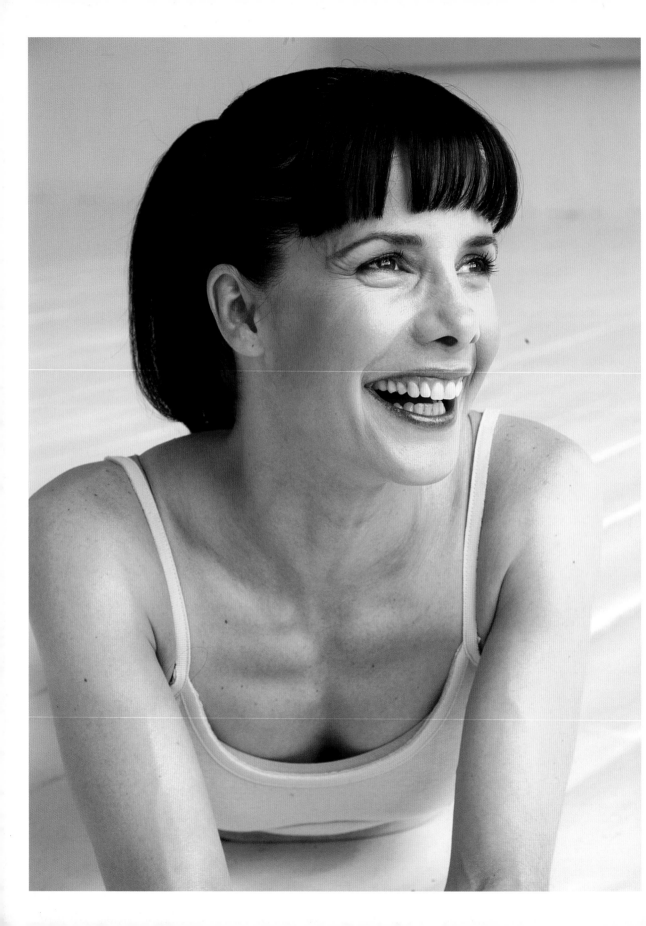

Healthy Living Tips

I am fanatical about what I eat otherwise I couldn't do what I do at my age, which means I eat well all the time. I rarely eat red meat and instead live on chicken, fish and brown rice (great for digestion), always eating more than five portions of fruit and vegetables a day.

I only eat pasta once a week and, apart from that, I stay off wheat completely. I eat rice and oat-based cereals and bananas to give me energy. I do have about three glasses of red wine a week because I know it's good for the heart, but I also make sure I drink plenty of water, especially as I am dancing all the time.

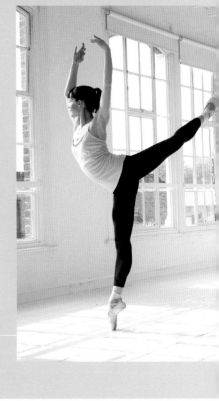

'I know now what's going to get me through a performance and what isn't and what's going to help my body recover from an injury and what's not'

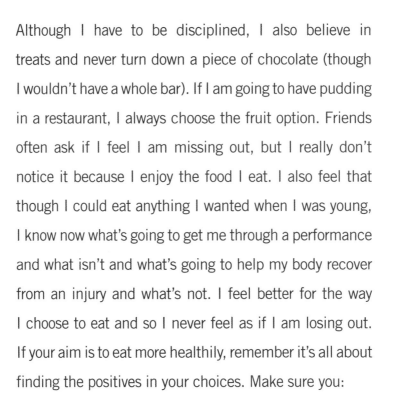

Although I have to be disciplined, I also believe in treats and never turn down a piece of chocolate (though I wouldn't have a whole bar). If I am going to have pudding in a restaurant, I always choose the fruit option. Friends often ask if I feel I am missing out, but I really don't notice it because I enjoy the food I eat. I also feel that though I could eat anything I wanted when I was young, I know now what's going to get me through a performance and what isn't and what's going to help my body recover from an injury and what's not. I feel better for the way I choose to eat and so I never feel as if I am losing out. If your aim is to eat more healthily, remember it's all about finding the positives in your choices. Make sure you:

Eat five portions of fruit and vegetables a day

Apples, bananas, lots of red berries and green leafy vegetables are particularly good because they are crammed full of vitamins and minerals and also add fibre to your diet.

Have a diet rich in calcium

Unless you're allergic to dairy, don't be tempted to ditch milk from your diet, because calcium is essential for strong bones. If you want to watch your weight, go for semi-skimmed, skimmed milk or soya milk because they contain exactly the same amount of calcium as the full-fat variety.

Eat protein

Include protein such as meat, fish and eggs, or tofu, chickpeas and soya (if you're a vegetarian) in your daily diet. About twenty-five percent of your daily food intake should come from protein because it's essential for building bones, muscles, healthy teeth, hair and nails. The best sources are chicken, fish, soya products, milk and eggs. A diet rich in protein (as opposed to a protein-only diet) will also control your appetite and stimulate your hormones to burn fat in the body.

Eat unsaturated fats

Also known as essential fatty acids, unsaturated fats (fats that are liquid at room temperature) are found in olive oil, salmon, tuna and sardines and are good for your heart health. This is why oily fish, which are rich in Omega-3 essential fatty acids, should be added to your diet three times a week for maximum benefits.

Drink more water

Research shows that one in five of us consume too little water throughout the day. The current recommendation is 1.5 litres (about eight to ten glasses) and not drinking this amount means most of us suffer from borderline dehydration, which leads to tiredness and a tendency to snack for energy. Water is also vital for optimum health, especially when you exercise. Not only does it hydrate organs and cushion the nervous system, but it also stops you reaching for food when what you really want is a drink (thirst receptors often get mixed up with hunger receptors).

Don't limit your carbohydrates

Eat less refined carbohydrates, such as white bread and pasta, white rice and potato, but do eat more wholemeal pasta, brown rice, wholemeal bread and green vegetables. It's a myth that dancers don't eat carbohydrates; in fact we need more of them because this is where we get the energy from for dancing. However, the average person doesn't need that many and should always eat carbohydrates earlier in the day because they are difficult to digest.

Think about your posture

Good posture is the key to having poise and confidence. This means it's important to always think about how you do everyday things, such as sitting, standing and bending. Never throw yourself into a chair when you sit down or brace yourself when you get up. Instead, focus on how you use your body before you do an action. By far the best way to do this is to always pull your bellybutton to your spine and imagine a string pulling you upwards from the top of your head when you walk, stand up or even bend down. The principles of the Pilates, floor barre and stretch workout will help you to make this action second nature, but to help maintain good posture make sure you do the following when:

Sitting

Never sit with your legs crossed because it twists your hips and pelvis. Sit with your legs in parallel and feet flat on the floor. Also, try to not slump into a chair, but instead sit out of your hips and support your back by drawing your stomach in slightly. Sitting on a stool can help you to work at this because you have no back support, but remember to sit so your bottom is to the back of the seat and to sit up out of your hips and not slump.

Standing

The best tip I was ever given for this is to relax your knees when you're standing so you're not standing back into them. If you look at yourself in a mirror side on, standing back into your knees causes an unnatural curve in your lower back. Stand with your knees slightly bent and your tailbone will drop down and your body will stand straighter. A good way of knowing if you're doing this correctly is to make sure your body weight is over your toes, not your heels. If your weight is settled into your heels, your shins will take the pressure and become tight and painful.

Walking

The only thing to remember here is to always walk with a heel-to-toe action (heel hits the ground first and rolls through to the toes), but don't walk like a dancer on your heels and with turned-out feet. I have to remind myself to walk heel to toe all the time to stop tendonitis happening because years of doing exercise in turnout has made me walk like this. It's always good to stretch your calves after a long walk.

Bending and carrying children

Firstly, never pitch forwards to pick a child up, always bend your knees, squat and reach forwards. It's the number one way to never hurt your back. Secondly, when carrying a child don't lean back with the weight against you or your hip; hold your stomach in and stand straight so the weight is balanced upwards, not backwards or to the side. Thirdly, use your arms. I always hold my younger daughter Zoe under her bottom and in front of me, and then bend my knees slightly to support myself when I am walking around with her. I've also learnt not to hunch forwards when carrying one of my children, all of which sounds fanatical, but it works. Finally, with two young daughters who get envious when I'm holding one over the other, I've also learnt that the only way to hold them both is to come down to their level, sit on the floor and hug them there. It saves me from being trampled on and from a backache.

Stay active

To stay healthy, it's recommended that you should take at least thirty minutes of physical activity five times a week. This is an activity that gets you breathing faster, increases your heart rate and warms you up. While the Pilates, floor barre and stretch workout works on improving muscle tone, cardiovascular exercise works on burning fat and keeping your heart healthy.

If you love dancing, this is good news because most dance styles, such as tap dancing and flamenco, are very energetic, but even a slow waltz is equivalent of at least a moderate (three miles per hour) walk. Anyone who does salsa or ballet will up their heart rate, warm up and breathe quickly. Apart from the obvious aerobic benefits to your heart and lungs, dance classes help increase muscle strength, promote flexibility and improve alignment and balance. Better still, the movements complement the Pilates, floor barre and stretch workout because they move your body in a range of diverse directions, which help tone and strengthen parts

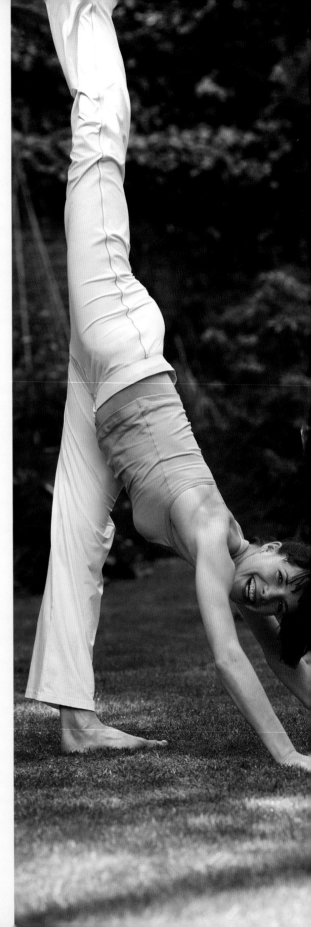

of the legs, stomach and back that are usually missed within a normal gym workout. The fat-burning quota of dancing is also higher than you may think, with the average person burning around three to ten calories a minute. This means a medium-paced salsa class could work off around 350 to 400 calories an hour, or basically your entire lunch! If dancing's not your thing, then other activities I love include:

Walking

This improves cardiovascular strength (the way your lungs and heart work) as well as muscle strength. Plus, it's cheap, it's easy and it can be done in high heels (good for calf strength)! Always walk with a heel-to-toe action and make sure you walk at a pace that makes your heart work that little bit faster. Walk every day for at least thirty minutes.

Swimming

This is an excellent form of exercise that I love. Like ballet, it uses all your muscles and improves upper and lower body strength, as well as aerobic strength. It's also cheap and easy to do, though be sure to push yourself and not just float and glide for thirty minutes a day. One good way is to swim ten lengths, and then use a paddle board and swim another ten, focusing on your legs. Swim for at least twenty minutes and change your activity each day, swimming perhaps front crawl one day, breaststroke the next and backstroke the following.

Cycling

This works the arms and legs and can be fun, though you need to do it for longer than the above to get the full benefit. Keep the seat high so the thighs don't get tight and bulky and don't rely on momentum to get you around, go at a steady pace. Always remember to stretch your thighs after cycling to stop them getting bulky.

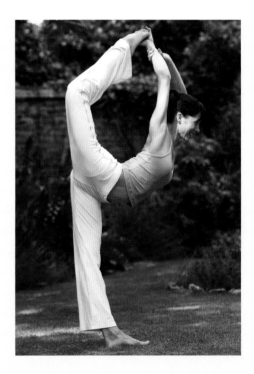

'While the Pilates, floor barre and stretch workout works on improving muscle tone, cardiovascular exercise works on burning fat and keeping your heart healthy'

GLOSSARY

Pilates

alignment
The body during every Pilates exercise should be in alignment. This means the joints of the body are always in line and symmetrical to each other.

core/centre
Every movement in Pilates initiates from the core. This is the band of muscles (the transversus abdominals and the diagonal obliques) that wraps around your body like a corset, helping to support you and give you good posture. Building strength here is essential for a healthy spine and the much-coveted flat stomach.

drawing in of the core
This is the bellybutton to spine movement, which basically engages your core muscles, pulls your pelvic floor up and helps you lift out of your waist.

glutes
Your bottom muscles that lie above your hamstrings.

hamstrings
The muscles that run down the back of your legs from your bottom to your knees.

lengthening
A feeling rather than a forced movement, whereby you imagine your neck slowly stretching away from your head or your leg stretching away from your hip.

momentum
A force of movement to get your body through a hard exercise. In Pilates, movement should not come from momentum, but from core strength to help build and tone muscle. The key is to control all movements and not rely on speed.

neutral spine
The position of your spine when you're standing or lying on the floor, shown by having a small natural curve to your lower back.

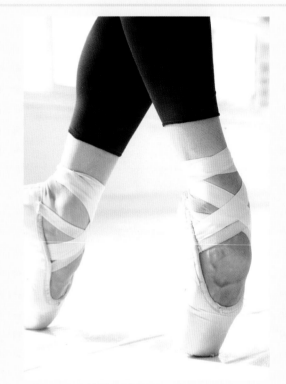

obliques
These are your side abdominal muscles, which lie around your waist.

quads
Front of the thigh muscles that run from your hip to your knee.

scooping
Pulling your bellybutton in towards your spine and, at the same time, imagining your stomach being scooped inwards and upwards.

shoulder stabilization
The sliding of your shoulder blades down your back to ensure that your shoulders are in the right position for an exercise (that is, not up around your ears).

Floor Barre and Standing Barre

adagio
A slow tempo, but in ballet it refers to a series of slow ballet moves.

à la seconde
A movement performed in second position.

à terre
A movement performed on the floor.

barre
A long horizontal bar that's attached to a wall. It is the place where dancers adapt the floor barre workout to a standing position to warm up every day.

centre floor
The centre of the room where exercises are danced without the aid of the barre.

cou-de-pied
A ballet position in which one foot is placed in front of the opposing ankle.

dégagé
A *tendu* in which the foot comes off the floor at a forty-five-degree angle.

demi-plié
Half a *plié*, where you bend your knees as far as you can while still keeping both heels planted on the ground.

devant
Meaning, literally, 'in front'.

développé
A slow unfolding of the leg so that you can extend it into the air.

en l'air
A movement in the air.

fondu
A one-legged knee bend.

frappé
A whipping/striking movement where you strike the floor or wall with your foot.

glissé
A movement of the foot where it slides along and off the floor.

grand battement
A high throwing kick.

grand plié
A deep knee bend in which heels can come off the floor.

pas
A step.

pirouette
A turn.

plié
A knee bend where you bend your knees while still keeping both heels planted on the ground.

port de bras
A 'carriage of the arms', this is a movement of the arms from one position to another.

relevé
A rise to the balls of the feet.

retiré
A move where a pointed foot is lifted and placed by the other knee (to look like a number four).

rond de jambe à terre
A semicircle drawn by the foot on the floor.

rond de jambe en l'air
A semicircle drawn by the foot in the air.

tendu
Means 'to brush' and is a brushing movement of the foot along the floor or wall.

tendu à la seconde
A brushing movement of the foot along the floor or wall to the side.

tendu derrière
A brushing movement of the foot along the floor behind you.

tendu devant
A brushing movement of the foot along the floor or wall in front of you.

turnout
Turning the legs out to ninety degrees from the hips.

BIOGRAPHY

Darcey Bussell was born in London on 27 April 1969. At the age of thirteen she was accepted into the Royal Ballet School where she studied for five years before joining Sadler's Wells Royal Ballet in 1987. In September 1988 Darcey joined the Royal Ballet, becoming a First Soloist; three months later she was promoted to Principal – a position she held until October 2006 when she became a Principal Guest Artist with the Royal Ballet. She has danced for the New York City Ballet, the Kirov Ballet of St. Petersburg and the La Scala Ballet Company of Milan, and has guested internationally with several other companies.

Darcey was awarded Dancer of the Year in 1990 by *Dance & Dancers* magazine. That same year she also received both the Sir James Garreras Award for the most promising newcomer and the Evening Standard Ballet Award. She was joint winner of the Cosmopolitan Achievement Award in the performing art category in 1991, and was made a Commander of the Order of the British Empire (CBE) in the 2006 Birthday Honours List.

Darcey and her husband, Angus, have two daughters, Phoebe and Zoe.

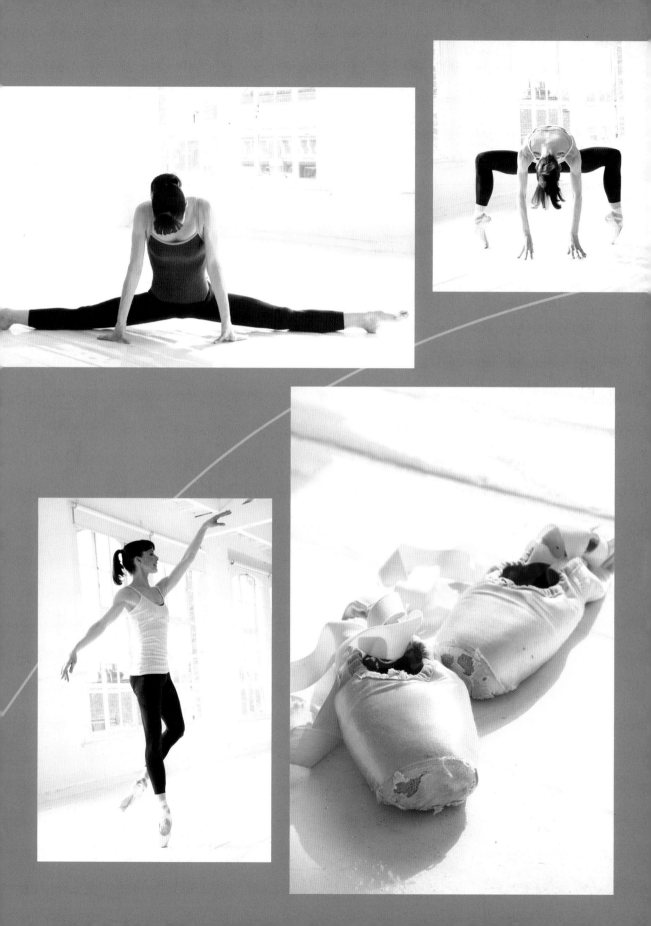

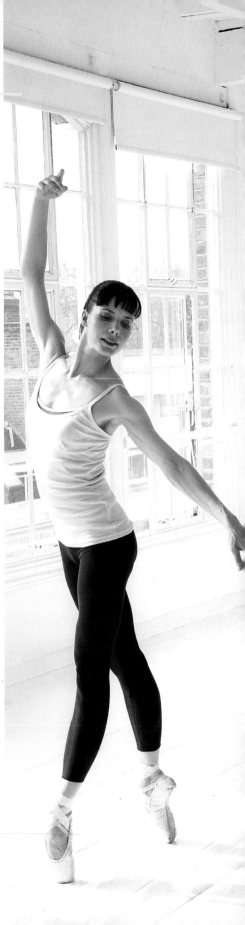

ACKNOWLEDGEMENTS

Thank you to the Royal Ballet, my colleagues and my friends for always reminding me that you never stop learning in life.

To the Penguin team, Chantal Gibbs, Kate Adams, Kate Brunt and Sarah Fraser, for knowing in advance all the floor barre positions and always being inspiring, and also to Anita Naik, a big thank you. To Clifford Bloxham and Sandy Lund at Octagon, and to Charlotte Toosey for keeping everyone in contact and smoothing the whole process.

To Shock Absorber and Nike for lending me the clothes for the book photography. To Iain Philpott, the photographer, for having such insight and professionalism and giving me great confidence.

To my family: my husband for being there every step of the way, and Phoebe and Zoe for making my life so real.